# Imaging Informatics for Healthcare Professionals

**Series Editors**
Peter M. A. van Ooijen, University Medical Center Groningen
University of Groningen, GRONINGEN, The Netherlands

Erik R. Ranschaert, Faculty of Medicine and Health Sciences
Ghent University, Ghent, Belgium

Annalisa Trianni, Department of Medical Physics, ASUIUD
UDINE, Italy

Michail E. Klontzas, Institute of Computer Science,
Foundation for Research and Technology (FORTH) and
University Hospital of Heraklion, Heraklion, Greece

The series Imaging Informatics for Healthcare Professionals is the ideal starting point for physicians and residents and students in radiology and nuclear medicine who wish to learn the basics in different areas of medical imaging informatics. Each volume is a short pocket-sized book that is designed for easy learning and reference.

The scope of the series is based on the Medical Imaging Informatics subsections of the European Society of Radiology (ESR) European Training Curriculum, as proposed by ESR and the European Society of Medical Imaging Informatics (EuSoMII). The series, which is endorsed by EuSoMII, will cover the curricula for Undergraduate Radiological Education and for the level I and II training programmes. The curriculum for the level III training programme will be covered at a later date. It will offer frequent updates as and when new topics arise.

Erik R. Ranschaert
Michail E. Klontzas
Nabile M. Safdar
Editors

# Sustainability of AI in Radiology

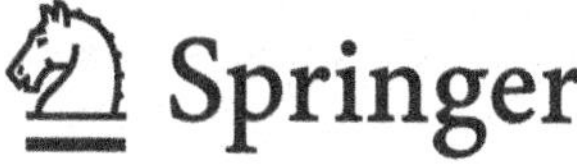

*Editors*
Erik R. Ranschaert
Faculty of Medicine and Health Sciences
Ghent University
Ghent, Belgium

Michail E. Klontzas
Department of Radiology, School of Medicine
University of Crete
Heraklion, Greece

Nabile M. Safdar
School of Medicine
Emory University
Atlanta, GA, USA

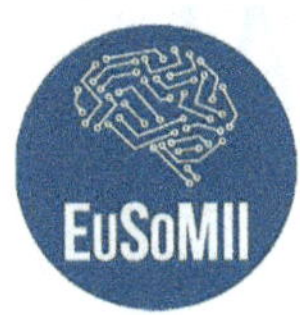


ISSN 2662-1541 ISSN 2662-155X (electronic)
Imaging Informatics for Healthcare Professionals
ISBN 978-3-032-15692-1 ISBN 978-3-032-15693-8 (eBook)
https://doi.org/10.1007/978-3-032-15693-8



This Springer imprint is published by the registered company Springer Nature Switzerland AG
The registered company address is: Gewerbestrasse 11, 6330 Cham, Switzerland

# Foreword

We live in an age frequently designated the Anthropocene, implying that the changes in our planet's environment are increasingly due to humanity's actions, rather than the geophysical forces which dominated previously. Climate change, species extinctions, food insecurity: all these factors are influenced by human behaviour. Industrialisation, globalisation, changing work patterns and energy demands all contribute to alterations in our biosphere, with effects which will radically alter how (and whether) we, and all the other life-forms with which we share our "pale blue dot", live and thrive in the coming decades and centuries.

As workers in the field of radiology, it's easy to believe that these global changes are a problem for someone else, or, at least, that we're not contributing to harm by doing our work. After all, radiology is of inestimable value in healthcare, with constantly developing capabilities and growing impact. However, despite its benefits, increasing imaging and interventional radiological utilisation results in significant environmental impacts. CT and MR imaging were estimated to contribute up to 0.77% of total global carbon dioxide emissions in 2016, with expected growth of 30% by 2030 (aviation contributed 2.5% in 2023) [1]. We find ourselves confronted with potentially competing imperatives: to optimise the benefit for individual patients and societies as a whole from using our radiological skills and resources, while minimising the potentially negative impact of utilisation of these skills and resources on our planetary environment. The dilemma is certainly not soluble by limiting utilisation; why should patients be denied potential immediate or short-term benefit from altruistically motivated healthcare in order to reduce the risk of a future more-nebulous planetary impact? Nonetheless, there are actions we in the radiology world can take to reduce our environmental impact without reducing provision of appropriate and necessary care, and new ways of thinking about resource allocation and utilisation among industry and end-users have the potential to mitigate environmental impacts caused by the practice of our specialty. Some of these are simple, and only require a heightening of our awareness of unnecessary energy use or wasteful consumption. Others are more complex, and need substantial manufacturing and design changes in equipment development.

Artificial Intelligence (AI) is a growing influence in daily life, not least in healthcare, and encompasses intrinsic impacts on greenhouse gas emissions and other environmental and societal consequences. These may be negative (e.g. in the context of energy utilisation, data centre construction and operation, etc.) or positive (e.g. more-efficient imaging data acquisition and transfer, lower-energy modes of operating equipment, etc.) [2]. Bearing in mind the imperative to always strive to help patients by utilising radiology [3], value delivery can be augmented by judicious use of these new tools. Furthermore, AI algorithms can be harnessed to find new, as-yet-unexplored means of improving efficacy of imaging and intervention, and to minimise unnecessary imaging.

This book, forming part of the series on Imaging Informatics for Healthcare Professionals, explores all these issues. Experts in the relevant fields detail and explain key aspects of sustainability as it relates to radiology, and how AI may influence these issues in the future. Energy efficiency, data management and societal and regulatory issues are all addressed, concluding with an overview of specific potential helpful actions and adaptations.

We are privileged to live and work in an era of rapidly expanding possibilities, both in the conduct of our radiological specialty, and in the tools which allow us serve our patients. Recent weather events, wildfires and population shifts can be traced to human impacts on our planet's health. As healthcare providers, we contribute to human well-being and see the effects of ill-health (and strive to eliminate or mitigate it). We can and should bring the same skills and focus to bear on planetary health, at least in so far as our specialty relates to it, positively and negatively. This book aims to guide readers to learn about how radiology and sustainability interact, and to point the way toward how we can harness AI and other tools to protect our planet, our patients and ourselves. Humanity has "sown the wind"; rather than "reaping the whirlwind", guides like this can teach us how to harvest a bountiful crop of benefit from that sowing.

Department of Radiology
University College Cork (UCC)
Cork, Ireland
4/11/25

Adrian P. Brady

## References

1. Rockall AG, Allen B, Brown MJ, El-Diasty T, Fletcher J, Gerson RF, Goergen S, Marrero González AP, Grist TM, Hanneman K, Hess CP, Ho ELM, Salama DH, Schoen J, Sheard S. Sustainability in radiology: position paper and call to action from ACR, AOSR, ASR, CAR, CIR, ESR, ESRNM, ISR, IS3R, RANZCR and RSNA. Eur Radiol. 2025;35:5427–36. https://doi.org/10.1007/s00330-025-11413-7
2. Kocak B, Ponsiglione A, Romeo V, Ugga L, Huisman M, Cuocolo R. Radiology AI and sustainability paradox: environmental economic dimensions. Insights Imaging. 2025;16:88. https://doi.org/10.1186/s13244-025-01962-2
3. Brady AP, Bello JA, Derchi LE, Fuchsjäger M, Goergen S, Krestin GP, Lee EJ, Levin DC, Pressaco J, Rao V, Slavotinek J, Visser JJ, Walker REA, Brink JA. Radiology in the era of value-based healthcare. A multi-society expert statement from the ACR, CAR, ESR, IS3R, RANZCR, and RSNA. Insights Imaging. 2020;11:136. https://doi.org/10.1186/s13244-020-00941-z

# Contents

# Introduction: Sustainability in Radiology and Healthcare

# 1

Erik R. Ranschaert, Michail E. Klontzas, and Nabile M. Safdar

The authors confirm that the conceptual figure (Fig. 1.1) within this chapter was generated with assistance from a large language model (LLM), specifically ChatGPT. This use case, which involves generative content creation rather than mere copy editing, is documented in accordance with the publisher's AI Authorship Policy, ensuring human accountability for the final figure design and content. The use of AI tools for figure generation is a practice where AI can be utilized without concerns regarding copyright, provided the application is properly documented.

E. R. Ranschaert (✉)
Faculty of Medicine and Health Sciences, Ghent University, Ghent, Belgium
e-mail: erik.ranschaert@ugent.be

M. E. Klontzas
School of Medicine, University of Crete, Rethymno, Greece
e-mail: miklontzas@uoc.gr

N. M. Safdar
Department of Radiology and Imaging Sciences, Emory University, Atlanta, GA, USA
e-mail: nabile.m.safdar@emory.edu



E. R. Ranschaert et al. (eds.), *Sustainability of AI in Radiology*, Imaging Informatics for Healthcare Professionals,
https://doi.org/10.1007/978-3-032-15693-8_1

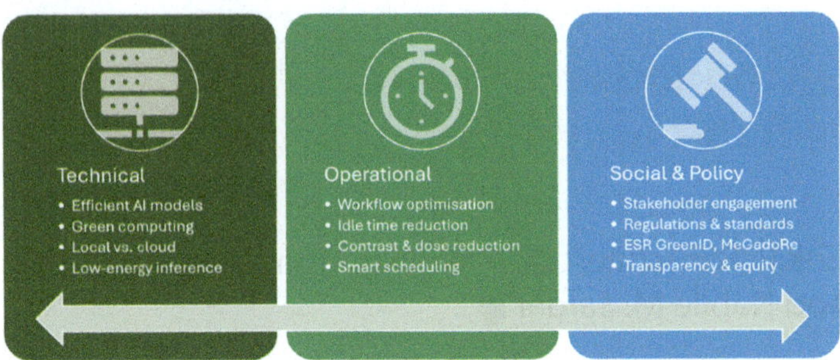


**Fig. 1.1** The three interconnected pillars of sustainable AI in radiology: (1) technical efficiency, (2) operational integration, and (3) social and regulatory alignment. (AI generated image created with Chat GPT, 2025)

## 1.1 Sustainability Challenges in Radiology

Healthcare systems worldwide are experiencing escalating demands driven by demographic shifts, notably aging populations, and the rising prevalence of chronic diseases, leading to increased reliance on medical imaging for diagnosis and treatment [1].

Although medical imaging substantially improves diagnostic accuracy and patient outcomes, its expanding usage contributes significantly to higher healthcare costs and increased energy consumption, thus posing notable environmental and economic challenges. Radiology departments are particularly energy-intensive, primarily due to MRI and CT scanners that rank among the highest energy-consuming medical technologies, significantly contributing to hospital-wide energy usage [2].

Recent research has revealed that radiology departments waste 40–91% of energy usage in nonproductive states, particularly when imaging machines remain powered on but idle [3] . Studies have also found that shutting down idle medical imaging devices can lead to significant energy savings, with estimated reductions of up to 72,337 kWh per year, equivalent to the energy consumption of 14 households [4]. Additionally, radiology generates significant material waste, particularly through single-use plastics, excessive packaging, and disposable items such as syringes, needles, biopsy instruments, and gloves. For instance, interventional radiology procedures generate substantial waste due to the extensive use of single-use plastics and packaging materials. An audit revealed that such procedures produce an average of 8 kg of waste per case, with coiling and embolization cases generating up to 13.1 kg and 10.3 kg, respectively [5]. Much of this plastic waste may fragment into microplastics, which can persist in the environment and enter aquatic and terrestrial ecosystems.

The extensive use of contrast agents further contributes to environmental contamination. Iodinated contrast media (ICM) and gadolinium-based contrast agents (GBCA), widely used in diagnostic procedures, accumulate in aquatic ecosystems through patient excretion. These agents often remain unmetabolized, leading to environmental contamination [6]. Research has confirmed the presence of these agents in surface water, groundwater, and drinking water in various regions worldwide, raising substantial concerns regarding environmental contamination [7].

Effective sustainability measures must therefore address both energy and material waste.

## 1.2 The Role of AI in Sustainable Radiology

The pressing sustainability challenges outlined above in Sect. 1.1 highlight the urgent need for systemic changes in how radiology is practiced and managed. While traditional strategies such as energy audits, equipment shutdown protocols, and waste segregation remain important, they are often limited in scope and scalability. Recent advances in artificial intelligence (AI) offer promising new tools to tackle these issues in a more dynamic and data-driven manner. By optimizing imaging workflows, minimizing resource use, and supporting decision-making, AI can act as a catalyst for more environmentally responsible radiology. The following sections explore how AI can actively contribute to sustainability, starting with its role in reducing energy consumption and material waste.

**Table 1.1** Overview of AI applications contributing to sustainability in radiology

| AI solution | Sustainability impact | Clinical or technical application |
|---|---|---|
| Automated imaging protocol selection | Reduces energy consumption, contrast media use, and waste | AI-driven CT and MRI protocol optimization based on clinical indication |
| AI-based image reconstruction | Reduces scan duration, energy use, and patient throughput | Deep learning algorithms in MRI and CT reconstruction |
| Imaging appropriateness support (pre-imaging CDS) | Decreases unnecessary imaging, thus reducing waste and resource use | AI tools for imaging appropriateness support (assessing necessity of imaging requests) |
| Predictive maintenance | Extends equipment lifespan, reduces material and electronic waste | AI systems predicting equipment maintenance needs |
| AI-assisted image analysis | Enhances diagnostic efficiency, reduces radiologist interpretation time | Automatic abnormality detection and analysis in MRI and CT and other modalities |
| Dose and contrast reduction | Minimizes radiation exposure and contrast agent usage | AI reconstruction algorithms reducing radiation dose and contrast volume |

Table 1.1 summarizes a range of AI applications currently used or under development in radiology and outlines their direct and indirect impacts on sustainability. These technologies are not only clinically valuable but are also critical enablers of greener radiological practices.

### 1.2.1 AI in Energy and Material Waste Reduction

AI significantly contributes to sustainability by optimizing imaging procedures to align with patient-specific and clinical needs. Automated protocol selection systems can reduce redundant scanning and help tailor CT and MRI parameters, which lead to lower radiation exposure and contrast usage [8, 9]. AI-powered dose modulation and contrast optimization techniques ensure that material consumption is minimized without compromising image quality [6].

AI-based image reconstruction technologies enable faster acquisitions, reducing scan times by 30–50% and lowering the energy demand of imaging equipment during each procedure [10]. This also improves patient comfort and scanner availability. Additionally, clinical decision support systems reduce the number of inappropriate imaging studies, conserving both energy and consumables [10].

Predictive maintenance systems, another application of AI, can forecast technical faults in imaging devices, preventing unplanned downtime and extending equipment lifespan. These tools help avoid premature replacements and reduce the environmental costs of equipment manufacturing and disposal.

### 1.2.2 Efficient Integration of AI in Radiology Infrastructure

While AI offers significant sustainability benefits in theory, realizing these advantages in clinical practice depends on how these tools are integrated into the hospital's digital and physical infrastructure. A major consideration is the choice between cloud-based and local deployment. Cloud-based AI offers scalability, centralized data processing, and enhanced collaboration, which can lead to streamlined workflows and operational cost savings [11]. However, continuous data transmission and remote processing can contribute to higher cumulative energy demands. Local deployment, on the other hand, requires a higher initial investment in hardware and setup, but allows for immediate data access, lower latency, and often reduced long-term energy usage [10].

At present, most radiology AI tools are built on specialized deep learning models that are trained to perform specific tasks such as lesion detection or protocol optimization. These task-specific models generally consume less energy and computational resources than generalized foundational models, which are larger, multipurpose systems trained on extensive and diverse datasets [12]. While foundational models may become more common in future radiology applications due to their flexibility, they currently remain energy-intensive and are not yet widely adopted.

To ensure sustainable AI implementation, healthcare institutions must evaluate their internal IT capacity, including storage, processing power, network bandwidth, and system interoperability. Integration with core systems such as Picture Archiving and Communication System (PACS) and Radiology Information System (RIS) is essential to support automated workflows and efficient data exchange. Robust data management strategies—such as optimized image compression and tiered storage—can further enhance sustainability outcomes [13].

### 1.2.3 Operational Efficiency and Workflow Optimization

Beyond technical capabilities, AI can also enhance the sustainability of radiology by streamlining departmental workflows. By reducing patient no-shows, eliminating duplicate imaging, and optimizing scanner scheduling and transport logistics, AI tools can improve patient throughput and resource efficiency. Smart injectors and advanced scheduling systems ensure optimal use of contrast agents and minimize waste during exam preparation [6]. These process-oriented interventions reduce not only environmental impact but also operational costs, supporting the broader institutional goal of delivering high-quality care in an efficient, sustainable manner.

### 1.2.4 Stakeholder Involvement and Collaboration

Sustainable radiology is not solely a technological endeavor—it requires institutional commitment and collaboration among diverse stakeholders. Radiologists, radiographers, clinical physicists, IT administrators, managers, equipment manufacturers, and patients each have a role to play. Establishing "green teams" within departments, promoting sustainability education, and sharing best practices across institutions can amplify the impact of technological interventions [6]. Professional societies also play a critical role by setting standards, advocating for certification systems, and providing platforms for collaboration and benchmarking. For instance, the European Society of Radiology (ESR) has introduced the GreenID Certification, a structured sustainability accreditation scheme for radiology departments. The initiative includes a staged certification process with bronze, silver, and gold levels based on performance in areas such as energy usage, waste management, procurement, and optimized imaging workflows. Its pilot phase involved 22 hospitals, demonstrating the practical feasibility and institutional value of embedding sustainability into daily radiology operations [14].

### 1.2.5 Balancing Benefits and Challenges of AI Integration

While AI offers numerous opportunities for sustainable radiology, it also introduces challenges—particularly related to energy consumption. Training large AI models can be extremely energy-intensive, especially for foundational models, which raises concerns about the carbon footprint of development cycles. It is essential to balance these upfront environmental costs against the long-term efficiency gains from clinical deployment [12]. Promoting green computing strategies—such as using renewable energy sources for training, optimizing code, and using efficient hardware—will be necessary to reduce the life cycle impact of AI in healthcare.

Taken together, the environmental, organizational, and ethical considerations discussed above reveal that sustainability in AI-driven radiology cannot be addressed in isolation. It requires alignment across technological innovation, system integration, and societal values. Figure 1.1 summarizes these three interconnected pillars that underpin sustainable AI in radiology.

## 1.3 Structure and Objectives of This Book

This book provides healthcare professionals and policymakers with strategies for integrating artificial intelligence into clinical practice. It is a core objective of the text to ensure that AI not only enhances patient care and operational efficiency but also contributes to long-term sustainability. The subsequent chapters delve into specific applications and their impact, illuminating AI's multifaceted potential while addressing critical considerations for its responsible and sustainable implementation.

Chapter 2 introduces the fundamental principles of artificial intelligence (AI) and its relevance to radiology. It explains different model architectures, including neural networks, transformers, and diffusion models, and provides a concise overview of how these models are trained, validated, and applied. The chapter also discusses the environmental impact of AI development and highlights key metrics for measuring its sustainability.

Chapter 3 examines sustainability in healthcare from a radiological perspective. It highlights the major contributors to environmental waste within imaging services, including energy use, single-use materials, and contrast agents. Examples from clinical practice illustrate how hospitals and departments can implement more sustainable radiology operations.

Chapter 4 focuses on the broader environmental footprint of radiology and investigates how AI can support more sustainable practices. Life cycle assessments of radiological equipment are presented, alongside analyses of how AI may contribute to resource optimization and smarter device utilization.

Chapter 5 provides an in-depth look at energy-efficient AI models and sustainable data practices. The chapter contrasts cloud-based with on-premises AI solutions and discusses model compression, data curation, and storage strategies that reduce carbon emissions and energy use. These insights are especially relevant for institutions planning long-term digital infrastructure.

Chapter 6 addresses the societal and ethical implications of AI-driven radiology. It explores the perspectives of patients, communities, and care providers, focusing on transparency, trust, access, and digital inclusivity. The authors advocate for inclusive development and public dialogue to ensure sustainable innovation aligns with societal values.

Chapter 7 reviews the regulatory and policy frameworks that govern sustainable AI in healthcare. It includes guidelines for green procurement, environmental certifications, and clinical safety compliance. This chapter is particularly useful for policymakers and institutional decision-makers.

Chapter 8 concludes the book by outlining a roadmap for the sustainable implementation of AI in radiology. The authors synthesize key themes and propose actionable strategies for long-term adoption, calling for collaboration across sectors and alignment with broader healthcare sustainability goals.

## 1.4 Conclusion

Radiology departments and imaging professionals are in a unique position to contribute to the global transition toward more sustainable healthcare. While AI offers powerful tools to reduce waste, improve efficiency, and support environmentally responsible practices, sustainability is not only about technology—it also requires cultural, organizational, and systemic change.

This introductory chapter sets the tone for a deeper exploration of how AI can support greener radiology, offering both practical insights and forward-looking reflections. Not every solution presented in this book is fully evidence-based—and it does not need to be. The aim is to stimulate awareness, share actionable ideas, and help radiology teams see where and how they can make a difference. By combining scientific insight with real-world experience, this book invites radiologists, hospital leaders, IT experts, and policy stakeholders to take meaningful steps toward more sustainable imaging.

## References


1. Smith-Bindman R, Kwan ML, Marlow EC, Theis MK, Bolch W, Cheng SY, Bowles EJA, Duncan JR, Greenlee RT, Kushi LH, Pole JD, Rahm AK, Stout NK, Weinmann S, Miglioretti DL. Trends in use of medical imaging in US health care systems and in Ontario, Canada, 2000-2016. JAMA. 2019;322:843–56. https://doi.org/10.1001/jama.2019.11456.
2. Heye T, Knoerl R, Wehrle T, Mangold D, Cerminara A, Loser M, Plumeyer M, Degen M, Lüthy R, Brodbeck D, Merkle E. The energy consumption of radiology: energy- and cost-saving opportunities for CT and MRI operation. Radiology. 2020;295:192084. https://doi.org/10.1148/radiol.2020192084.
3. Roletto A, Zanardo M, Bonfitto GR, Catania D, Sardanelli F, Zanoni S. The environmental impact of energy consumption and carbon emissions in radiology departments: a systematic review. Eur Radiol Exp. 2024;8:35. https://doi.org/10.1186/s41747-024-00424-6.
4. Heye T, Meyer MT, Merkle EM, Vosshenrich J. Turn it off! A simple method to save energy and CO 2 emissions in a hospital setting with focus on radiology by monitoring nonproductive energy-consuming devices. Radiology. 2023;307:e230162. https://doi.org/10.1148/radiol.230162.
5. Woolen SA, Kim CJ, Hernandez AM, Becker A, Martin AJ, Kuoy E, Pevec WC, Tutton S. Radiology environmental impact: what is known and how can we improve? Acad Radiol. 2023;30:625–30. https://doi.org/10.1016/j.acra.2022.10.021.
6. Dekker HM, Stroomberg GJ, Prokop M. Tackling the increasing contamination of the water supply by iodinated contrast media. Insights Imaging. 2022;13:30. https://doi.org/10.1186/s13244-022-01175-x.
7. Sengar A, Vijayanandan A. Comprehensive review on iodinated X-ray contrast media: complete fate, occurrence, and formation of disinfection byproducts. Sci Total Environ. 2021;769:144846. https://doi.org/10.1016/j.scitotenv.2020.144846.
8. Ahmadzade M, Moron FE, Shastri R, Lincoln C, Rad MG. AI-assisted post contrast brain MRI: eighty percent reduction in contrast dose. Acad Radiol. 2024; https://doi.org/10.1016/j.acra.2024.10.026.
9. McCollough CH, Leng S. Use of artificial intelligence in computed tomography dose optimisation. Ann ICRP. 2020;49:113–25. https://doi.org/10.1177/0146645320940827.
10. Doo FX, Vosshenrich J, Cook TS, Moy L, Almeida EPRP, Woolen SA, Gichoya JW, Heye T, Hanneman K. Environmental sustainability and AI in radiology: a double-edged sword. Radiology. 2024;310:e232030. https://doi.org/10.1148/radiol.232030.

11. Panner M. How the convergence of AI and the cloud can unlock breakthroughs and cost Savings in Radiology. Diagn Imaging. 2024;
12. Truhn D, Müller-Franzes G, Kather JN. The ecological footprint of medical AI. Eur Radiol. 2024;34:1176–8. https://doi.org/10.1007/s00330-023-10123-2.
13. Chartrand G, Cheng PM, Vorontsov E, Drozdzal M, Turcotte S, Pal CJ, Kadoury S, Tang A. Deep learning: a primer for radiologists. Radiographics. 2017;37:2113–31. https://doi.org/10.1148/rg.2017170077.
14. HealthManagement.org. Guiding Radiology to a Greener Future. https://healthmanagement.org/c/imaging/News/guiding-radiology-to-a-greener-future. 2025

# 2 Introduction to AI and Its Applications

Vicente Grau

## 2.1 Introduction

Artificial intelligence (AI) has experienced extraordinary success in recent years. It has affected virtually every sector of the economy, with the promise of increased productivity, new opportunities for growth, and novel application areas. This certainly includes healthcare, where AI developments are rapidly making their way in multiple applications, from drug development to risk prediction, diagnostics, or patient management. With AI showing particularly strong potential in image-related tasks, radiology is a natural application area, and as such it has already provided some of the most impactful early application cases. However, together with AI's immense promise, significant challenges arise. One of the most pressing is its impact on sustainability in healthcare: state-of-the-art AI methods require substantial computational resources. On the other hand, appropriate use of AI methods could reduce the environmental impact of healthcare. Detailed analysis and consideration of both positive and negative impacts will be fundamental on our way to a net zero carbon footprint in healthcare.

V. Grau (✉)
Institute of Biomedical Engineering, Department of Engineering Science, University of Oxford, Oxford, UK
e-mail: Vicente.grau@eng.ox.ac.uk





E. R. Ranschaert et al. (eds.), *Sustainability of AI in Radiology*, Imaging Informatics for Healthcare Professionals,
https://doi.org/10.1007/978-3-032-15693-8_2

## 2.2 Basics of AI

The modern concept of artificial intelligence (AI) has a long history, with developments evolving in parallel with the origins of computers in the mid-twentieth century [1]. However, it is only recently that it has experienced extraordinary success. Several factors have been instrumental; among them, we can mention:

- Rapid increases in computational performance; in particular, the availability of relatively inexpensive graphical processing units (GPUs), with their parallel processing capabilities
- The availability of large quantities of data from multiple sources across the Internet, many of them publicly accessible
- The development of novel mathematical algorithms, able to process information from such large amounts of data in an efficient way

The most prominent recent successes in AI have come from the subarea of machine learning (ML). While the terms ML and AI are sometimes used interchangeably, ML is a subset of AI in which algorithms learn directly from data without the explicit introduction of external rules. Deep learning (DL) is, in turn, a subset of ML. DL algorithms use Artificial Neural Networks (ANNs), with multiple layers sequentially connected, forming a "deep" structure.

## 2.3 Artificial Neural Networks: The Basis of Modern AI

While multiple architectures exist in modern AI, ANNs have been undoubtedly one of the main driving forces behind the recent success of the technology. ANNs are loosely inspired by the structure of the human brain. Individual *neurons* perform simple, nonlinear mathematical operations on their inputs, producing outputs that in turn form the input to other neurons. These mathematical operations contain a number of trainable *weights*, which are adjusted during training to perform a predefined task. The accuracy with which the task is performed is quantified by a *loss function*.

Neurons are typically structured in layers, with the outputs of each layer connected to the input of the next. In this way, one can create a multilayer perceptron (MLP), one of the key building blocks of deep neural networks. MLPs are formed by an input layer, an output layer, and one or more hidden layers. Neuron outputs are a function of their inputs, controlled by a set of tunable parameters (weights). These parameters are iteratively adjusted during training, with the objective of minimising the loss function. This is the way in which networks "learn" to perform specific tasks.

## 2.4 The Training Process: Training, Validation, and Test Sets

When training a neural network, the available data is divided into different subsets. The training set is used to calculate the optimal weights, i.e. the ones that produce a result as close as possible to the ground truth, as quantified by the loss function. Training is performed in an iterative way and measured in *epochs*; each time the network sees all the training data is counted as one epoch.

The validation set is used to estimate how well the network will perform on unseen data. This is important because of the risk of overfitting, i.e. obtaining a network that performs much better on the training set than on new data. To avoid this and optimise the network hyperparameters, during training, the model is periodically tested on the validation set. If the performance on the validation set starts to degrade, the training process can be stopped.

Finally, the test set is used as a final evaluation of the performance of the network. It must be used once the training process is fully completed and reflects how well the model will work when deployed in the real world (at least as long as the test set is representative of real-world scenarios).

When dealing with a limited number of samples (as is often the case in medical, and especially in radiological, applications), this split might not be the best use of the available data. A common alternative used in machine learning is n-fold cross-validation. Here the whole dataset is split into n "folds." The network is trained n times, each time using n-1 folds to train and the remaining fold to test. This provides a more robust metric of model accuracy at the expense of a substantial increase in computational training cost.

## 2.5 Supervised vs Unsupervised Learning

In applications such as disease detection or risk prediction, the most common approach is supervised learning. In supervised learning, the training dataset is fully annotated, i.e. there is a known "ground truth" for each data sample. This can be based on a separate test (e.g. a histopathology confirmation of a tumour in a radiological image) or assigned by an expert. The availability of ground truth allows the loss function to be defined as a direct, quantitative evaluation of the prediction accuracy.

In contrast, unsupervised (self-supervised) learning does not rely on annotations. In this case, the aim of the training process is to find the hidden structure of the data. For example, it can identify clusters (subgroups that share similar characteristics) in a group of patients, suggesting avenues for further investigation of physiological mechanisms.

Annotating medical data is expensive, and it is often difficult to obtain sufficiently large annotated datasets for fully supervised learning. An interesting alternative is semi-supervised learning, which uses a mixture of annotated and non-annotated data (which is easier to get in large numbers). The model can then learn by introducing the hidden structure of the unlabelled data while leveraging the ground truth available for the labelled data.

A recent advance that could have a sizeable impact on medical AI is the development of foundation models. Foundation models are trained on massive amounts of data, usually in a self-supervised way, with the objective of building a model that can adapt to many downstream tasks. They can then be fine-tuned to specific applications, often requiring only a fraction of the data that would be required if training the model from scratch.

## 2.6 Convolutional Neural Networks (CNNs) and Transformers

A typical characteristic of basic ANNs like the multilayer perceptron (MLP) is that they are fully connected, i.e. neurons in one layer connect to all neurons in adjacent layers. This is not particularly efficient in image analysis, where relationships between neighbouring pixels should generally carry a different weight to those between distant ones. CNNs (Fig. 2.1) exploit this idea by using convolutional layers, which combine spatially adjacent values through convolutional operations, calculating relevant patterns (features) such as edges, lines, or corners. Convolutional layers are combined with pooling layers, which downsample the feature maps. This structure is repeated a number of times; by gradually reducing the number of features, each one of them cov-

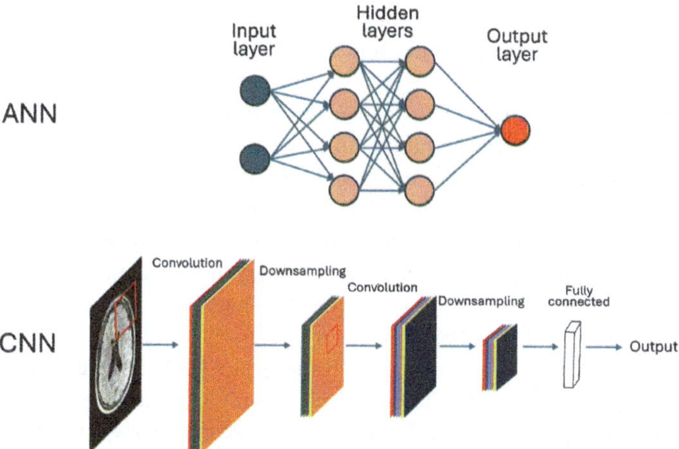


**Fig. 2.1** Comparison between ANN and CNN architectures. ANNs are typically fully connected, with each neuron connected to all others in adjacent layers. Each arrow in the ANN represents a weight, i.e. a trainable value. In contrast, in the CNN, the trainable values are those in convolution kernels, which combine adjacent pixels to generate multiple feature maps. These feature maps are progressively reduced in size up to the final fully connected layer

ers increasingly large image areas, allowing relationships to be calculated over increasingly large neighbourhoods. Typically, the last layer would be a fully connected one, combining the information from the whole image into a final value (e.g. a diagnostic label, or a risk value). Following developments like LeNet or AlexNet [2, 3], CNNs quickly became state of the art in image classification, including diagnosis and risk prediction in medical imaging.

Standard CNNs take an image as an input but output a single number, such as a classification label (e.g. normal/abnormal) or a quantification of risk based on the image contents. However, many imaging applications aim at transforming the original image into another image of the same size. A particularly important application in radiology is image segmentation, which can be achieved by transforming each pixel in an image into a label, corresponding to the organ or anatomical structure it belongs to. This was initially attempted by adding an expansive path or decoder at the end of CNN's contracting path or encoder. However, in this bottleneck architecture, the fine details of the original image are lost in the decoding process (which decreases the resolution), relying on the decoder to recover high-resolution details from a low-resolution representation. In practice, this tends to produce simplified segmentations missing finer details. A new architecture was proposed in [4]: the U-Net, which adds shortcuts (skip connections) connecting encoder layers to corresponding decoder ones. U-Nets showed remarkable accuracy and robustness to limited training data, quickly becoming the state of the art in medical image segmentation [5].

Another application for which the basic ANN architecture is not particularly well suited is the processing of sequences, where elements appear in a specific order. This is particularly relevant in Natural Language Processing (NLP). Initial attempts including architectures such as Recurrent Neural Networks achieved some success, but the combination of short- and long-range dependencies proved challenging. This led to one of the most important developments in AI in recent years: the Transformer architecture (Fig. 2.2). First proposed in the seminal paper "Attention is All You Need" [6], Transformers rely solely on a mechanism called

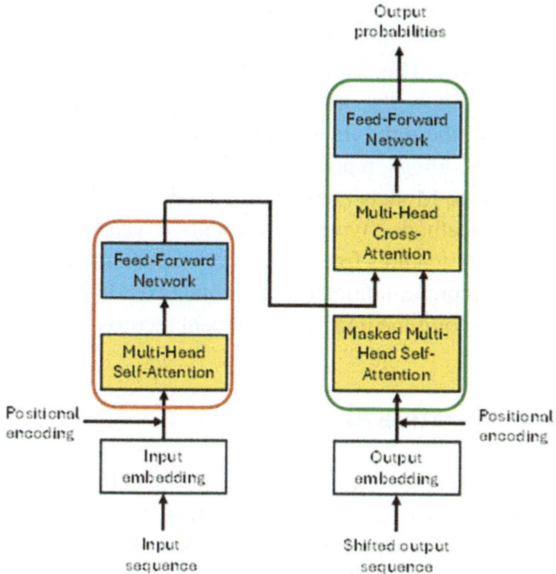


**Fig. 2.2** Basic Transformer architecture. On the left, the input sequence is position encoded and passed as input to the encoder. On the right, the decoder uses previously generated items (fed in as a shifted sequence), together with the input, to generate the output sequence

self-attention. Transformers are used to generate an output sequence from an input sequence using an encoder-decoder structure, combining multi-head self-attention and feed-forward networks. Instead of learning the position of each element (e.g. a word, in NLP) directly from the input sequence, Transformers use positional encoding vectors, which are added to word representations (embeddings). Positional encodings are typically calculated using sine and cosine functions, allowing the model to capture short- and long-range dependencies. Transformers have made possible the explosion in NLP in the last years, fuelled by Large Language models (LLMs) such as GPT [7]. The availability of effective AI tools for text processing opens up new, exciting opportunities for the use of AI in medicine; one of them involves generation and/or analysis of radiological reports [8].

While Transformers were not originally designed for image processing, their success encouraged researchers to explore their application in this area. This led to the concept of Vision Transformers (ViTs) [9]. To allow the application of Transformers on images, ViTs transform the input image into a sequence of image patches, including embeddings representing their location in the image. Visual Language Models combine the model capabilities of computer vision methods (typically through a vision encoder that extracts relevant features from images or videos) and LLMs to provide a shared representation of images and texts. In radiology, they can be used to combine images and patient records [10].

## 2.7 Generative AI

Much of the recent excitement about the capabilities of AI has come from the area of Generative AI, which aims at generating new samples based on patterns learned during training. One of the first successful approaches was the Variational Autoencoder (VAE) [11]. VAEs rely on an encoder-decoder architecture, much like others we have seen before in this chapter. The bottleneck between the encoder and the decoder contains a "compressed" (lower-dimensional) representation of the input; this "latent space" representation contains all the information necessary to generate the output image. In the original application, this output image is the same as the input (hence the name Autoencoder), but this can be generalized to produce transformed versions. The characteristic that allows VAEs to be used in a generative manner is that they learn a probability distribution (typically a Gaussian) over the latent space, thus allowing to sample this latent space to generate new outputs. VAEs have been shown to be useful in multiple medical imaging applications, including the generation of synthetic datasets (addressing the issue of data scarcity), denoising, image reconstruction, or detection of abnormalities in images [12]. However, they tend to produce less sharp images that may thus not appear as fully realistic.

Another fundamental method in Generative AI is the Generative Adversarial Network (GAN) [13]. GANs consist of two neural networks, a Generator and a Discriminator, which compete against each other. The Generator tries to produce samples (e.g. images) that look as much as possible like those in the training dataset, while the Discriminator tries to discern which samples are real and which are generated. During training, both networks become progressively better at their respective jobs. The final aim is for the Generator to become so good as to produce samples indistinguishable from the real ones.

GANs can also be used for image-to-image transformation. This was pioneered by the pix2pix approach [14], in which the discriminator has access to both input and output images, assessing their realism as a pair. The original pix2pix paper demonstrated the approach in multiple cases, e.g. transforming black-and-white to colour pictures, day to night photographs, or line sketches to fully formed images. This was swiftly followed by multiple users finding additional applications, from arts to medicine. However, the original GAN architecture requires paired samples (i.e. both the original and the transformed image) for training. This can be solved with the Cycle-GAN architecture [15], which adds a cycle consistency term voiding the requirement for image pairs during training.

While VAEs and GANs are still being applied in many areas, the current state of the art in photo-realistic image generation are Diffusion models [16]. Noise is gradually added to an original image, until it becomes indistinguishable from random noise. The Diffusion model is then trained to perform the inverse operation, going from random noise to a realistic image. Once trained, the model can be used to generate new images from random inputs. Recent models such as Stable Diffusion [17] can be conditioned using additional cues, such as text inputs or masks, allowing the generation of synthesised images with the desired characteristics and exceptional realism. An important limitation of Diffusion models is their large computational cost, both because of their complexity and need for large datasets for training.

## 2.8 AI in Radiology

Deep learning has shown great promise in radiology. Its applications range from image acquisition to analysis and include automating tasks to alleviate radiologists' workloads (e.g. segmentation, abnormality detection, measurement of anatomical structures) as well as extracting new biomarkers of clinical importance.

Following the strength of initial results in computer vision tasks such as the ImageNet Large Scale Visual Recognition (LSVR) challenge, image recognition and classification were identified as natural objectives for the application of AI in radiology. The same ideas that allowed image classification in the LSVR challenge can be applied to classify images into normal or pathological. For example, a method to detect chest CT scans containing tumours showed a performance comparable to human experts in [18]. One step forward from classification is for the networks to not just detect that an image is abnormal, but to detect the location of the abnormality. Following the same ideas, object detection and identification methods have also achieved remarkable accuracy.

An area in which progress has been particularly impressive is medical image segmentation. Manual segmentation is notoriously time-consuming, especially if 3D structures are to be segmented requiring slice-by-slice delineation of anatomical structures. The U-Net quickly became state of the art in automated medical image segmentation. In applications where a sufficient number of images is available, U-Nets have shown performance similar to that of human segmenters, as shown e.g. in the segmentation of cardiac MRI images in the UK Biobank [19]. One challenge of U-Nets is the need to adjust hyperparameters (e.g. the architecture of the network) to obtain optimal results. The no-new U-Net (nnUNet) [20] attempted to solve this problem by introducing an additional training process to estimate optimal hyperparameters, obtaining state-of-the-art results in a number of public segmentation challenges.

Image registration, i.e. the calculation of the spatial transformations required to align images to each other, is another long-standing challenge in medical imaging. While the application of deep learning to registration is not as straightforward as to image classification or segmentation, good progress has also been made, with methods that achieve state-of-the-art accuracy in a fraction of the time required by traditional methods [21].

Another area where initial results have shown remarkable promise is image-to-image transformation. Generative models can transform from one image "style" to a different one. This has been used to convert between imaging modalities (e.g. between CT and MRI) or to generate synthetic contrast images from non-contrast scans [22], promising a reduction to scanning costs and times and an improvement of patients' experience.

The success of AI in radiology has been significantly aided by the availability of large, publicly available imaging datasets. Following the success of foundation models in other areas, we have witnessed similar efforts in radiology. With the strength shown by LLMs, an obvious application is the generation and interpretation of radiological reports. Models can automatically generate reports from images or summarise them [23, 24]. Apart from text-related applications, foundation models have been developed for image analysis tasks. The Segment Anything Model (SAM) has been adapted to medical imaging with promising results [25]. Recently, foundation models have been trained and made available for different modalities, e.g. echocardiography [26].

## 2.9 The Environmental Impact of AI in Radiology

Globally, healthcare has been estimated to account for 5–8% of greenhouse gas emissions, with wealthier countries contributing at a disproportionate rate [27]. On its own, medical imaging may contribute up to 1% of global carbon footprint, with most of this contribution arising from manufacturing and powering up radiological equipment though AI is starting to have an important contribution of its own [28, 29]. The advent of AI and its impact on radiology has been characterized as a "double-edged sword" when accounting for its environmental effects [30]. Several potential positive impacts have been highlighted. By allowing high-quality reconstructions from shorter acquisitions, scanning times can be reduced [31]. In a similar way, AI could allow a reduction of radiation doses in CT without compromising image quality

[32]. AI can be used to determine the need for additional scans, reducing the resources allocated to "low-value imaging" [33, 34]. AI can help maximise efficiency by reducing scanner idle times, reducing the number of patient visits and minimising no-shows [35]. Exogenous contrast agents represent an important environmental impact of medical imaging procedures. AI-generated contrast has been proposed as a way to minimise contrast agent use, partially replacing gadolinium-based agents in MRI [36], or iodine-based ones in CT [37]. Similarly to MRI and CT, Positron Emission Tomography (PET) scans can be synthetically generated using AI [38].

On the negative side, with new models requiring increasing amounts of power for training and deployment, the environmental footprint of AI is a growing concern. The computational cost of new AI research has increased 300,000 times in recent years, leading to an enormous carbon footprint ("Red AI"). An alternative concept ("Green AI") has been proposed [39], which treats efficiency as a fundamental aspect of AI evaluation. The environmental impact of AI manifests in multiple ways. Training large models uses a large amount of energy: a single training run can cost as much as the daily carbon footprint of eight million people worldwide [40]. At inference (i.e. when running the model after it has been trained), the individual cost is much lower, but given that each model can be run millions of times, inference costs can quickly become larger than those of training. Data are typically kept in cloud-based storage, with its own environmental impact: globally, data centers may contribute to up to 2% of total electricity usage [41]. AI equipment becomes obsolete at a high rate, contributing to electronic waste. Finally, cooling of AI hardware requires substantial amounts of water.

To achieve the goals of Green AI in radiology, multiple interventions are needed. The environmental impact of AI methods should become an integral part of their assessment, together with currently used ones such as model accuracy. This requires impact calculation tools: while such have started to appear for general deep learning models [42]; they are not specifically adapted to radiology yet. Models should be chosen with the minimal computational footprint that solves the target application, rather than using the largest available models by default. Particular attention should be given to energy sources and geographical locations, favouring renewable sources and colder climates for hardware cooling. These interventions will require a combination of research and regulation in the foreseeable future.

## 2.10 Conclusion

AI is already revolutionizing radiology, improving accuracy, consistency, and efficiency of multiple radiological applications. However, its environmental footprint is many times overlooked. In the path towards net zero, the adoption of novel AI tools in radiology should be accompanied by an analysis of the balance of their environmental impacts.

## References


1. Xu Y, Liu X, Cao X, Huang C, Liu E, Qian S, et al. Artificial intelligence: a powerful paradigm for scientific research. Innovation [Internet]. 2021;2(4):100179. [cited 2025 Jul 18]; Available from: https://www.cell.com/action/showFullText?pii=S2666675821001041
2. Lecun Y, Bottou L, Bengio Y, Haffner P. Gradient-based learning applied to document recognition. Proc IEEE. 1998;86(11):2278–324.
3. Krizhevsky A, Sutskever I, Hinton GE. ImageNet classification with deep convolutional neural networks [Internet]. Available from: http://code.google.com/p/cuda-convnet/
4. Ronneberger O, Fischer P, Brox T. U-Net: convolutional networks for biomedical image segmentation. In: International Conference on Medical image computing and computer-assisted intervention. Cham: Springer; 2015. p. 234–41.
5. Isensee F, Jaeger PF, Kohl SAA, Petersen J, Maier-Hein KH. nnU-net: a self-configuring method for deep learning-based biomedical image segmentation. Nat Methods [Internet]. 2021;18(2):203–11. [cited 2025 Jul 18; Available from: https://www.nature.com/articles/s41592-020-01008-z
6. Vaswani A, Shazeer N, Parmar N, Uszkoreit J, Jones L, Gomez AN, et al. Attention is all you need. Adv Neural Inf Process Syst. 2017;30

7. Brown TB, Mann B, Ryder N, Subbiah M, Kaplan J, Dhariwal P, et al. Language models are few-shot learners [Internet]. 2020.. Available from: https://commoncrawl.org/the-data/
8. Casey A, Davidson E, Poon M, Dong H, Duma D, Grivas A, et al. A systematic review of natural language processing applied to radiology reports. BMC Med Inform Decis Mak. 2021;21:1. [Internet]. 2021 Jun 3 [cited 2025 Jul 18]; 21(1):1–18. Available from: https://bmcmedinformdecismak.biomedcentral.com/articles/10.1186/s12911-021-01533-7
9. Dosovitskiy A, Beyer L, Kolesnikov A, Weissenborn D, Zhai X, Unterthiner T, et al. An image is worth 16x16 words: transformers for image recognition at scale. In: ICLR 2021—9th International Conference on Learning Representations [Internet]; 2020. [cited 2025 Jul 10]; Available from: https://arxiv.org/pdf/2010.11929.
10. Azad R, Kazerouni A, Heidari M, Aghdam EK, Molaei A, Jia Y, et al. Advances in medical image analysis with vision transformers: a comprehensive review. Med Image Anal [Internet]. 2024;91:103000. [cited 2025 Jul 18]; Available from: https://www.sciencedirect.com/science/article/pii/S1361841523002608
11. Kingma DP, Welling M. Auto-encoding variational Bayes. In: 2nd International Conference on Learning Representations, ICLR 2014—Conference Track Proceedings [Internet]; 2013. [cited 2025 Jul 10]; Available from: https://arxiv.org/pdf/1312.6114.
12. Ehrhardt J, Wilms M. Autoencoders and variational autoencoders in medical image analysis. In: Biomedical image synthesis and simulation: methods and applications [Internet]; 2022. [cited 2025 Aug 9]; 129–62. Available from: https://www.sciencedirect.com/science/article/pii/B9780128243497000153.
13. Goodfellow IJ, Pouget-Abadie J, Mirza M, Xu B, Warde-Farley D, Ozair S, et al. Generative Adversarial Nets. Adv Neural Inf Process Syst [Internet]. 2014;27. [cited 2025 Aug 9]; Available from: http://www.github.com/goodfeli/adversarial
14. Isola P, Zhu JY, Zhou T, Efros AA, Research BA. Image-to-image translation with conditional adversarial networks [Internet]. 2017 . p. 1125–1134.. [cited 2025 Aug 7]. Available from: https://github.com/phillipi/pix2pix.
15. Zhu JY, Park T, Isola P, Efros AA. Unpaired image-to-image translation using cycle-consistent adversarial networks. In: Proceedings of the IEEE International Conference on Computer Vision [Internet]; 2017. p. 2242–51. [cited 2025 Jul 18]; 2017-October. Available from: https://arxiv.org/pdf/1703.10593.
16. Ho J, Jain A, Abbeel P. Denoising diffusion probabilistic models. Adv Neural Inf Process Syst [Internet]. 2020; [cited 2025 Jul 10]; 2020-December. Available from: https://arxiv.org/pdf/2006.11239
17. Rombach R, Blattmann A, Lorenz D, Esser P, Ommer B. High-resolution image synthesis with latent diffusion models. In: Proceedings of the IEEE

Computer Society Conference on Computer Vision and Pattern Recognition [Internet]; 2021. p. 10674–85. [cited 2025 Jul 10]; 2022-June. Available from: https://arxiv.org/pdf/2112.10752.

18. Ardila D, Kiraly AP, Bharadwaj S, Choi B, Reicher JJ, Peng L, et al. End-to-end lung cancer screening with three-dimensional deep learning on low-dose chest computed tomography. Nat Med [Internet]. 2019;25(6):954–61. [cited 2025 Jul 10]; Available from: https://pubmed.ncbi.nlm.nih.gov/31110349/
19. Bai W, Sinclair M, Tarroni G, Oktay O, Rajchl M, Vaillant G, et al. Automated cardiovascular magnetic resonance image analysis with fully convolutional networks 08 information and computing sciences 0801 artificial intelligence and image processing. J Cardiovasc Magn Reson [Internet]. 2018;20(1):1–12. [cited 2025 Jul 10]; Available from: https://jcmr-online.biomedcentral.com/articles/10.1186/s12968-018-0471-x
20. Isensee F, Jaeger PF, Kohl SAA, Petersen J, Maier-Hein KH. nnU-Net: a self-configuring method for deep learning-based biomedical image segmentation. Nat Methods [Internet]. 2021;18(2):203–11. [cited 2025 Jul 10]; Available from: https://www.nature.com/articles/s41592-020-01008-z
21. Chen J, Liu Y, Wei S, Bian Z, Subramanian S, Carass A, et al. A survey on deep learning in medical image registration: new technologies, uncertainty, evaluation metrics, and beyond. Med Image Anal [Internet]. 2025;100:103385. [cited 2025 Jul 10]; Available from: https://www.sciencedirect.com/science/article/pii/S1361841524003104
22. Chandrashekar A, Handa A, Shivakumar N, Lapolla P, Grau V, Lee R. A deep learning approach to generate contrast-enhanced computerised tomography angiography without the use of intravenous contrast agents. arXiv. 2020;
23. Tu T, Azizi S, Driess D, Schaekermann M, Amin M, Chang PC, et al. Towards generalist biomedical AI. NEJM AI. 2024;1(3)
24. Paschali M, Chen Z, Blankemeier L, Varma M, Youssef A, Bluethgen C, et al. Foundation models in radiology: what, how, why, and why not. Radiology. Radiological Society of North America Inc. 2025;314
25. Huang Y, Yang X, Liu L, Zhou H, Chang A, Zhou X, et al. Segment anything model for medical images? Med Image Anal [Internet]. 2024;92:103061. [cited 2025 Aug 7]; Available from: https://www.sciencedirect.com/science/article/abs/pii/S1361841523003213
26. Kim S, Jin P, Song S, Chen C, Li Y, Ren H, et al. EchoFM: foundation model for generalizable echocardiogram analysis. IEEE Trans Med Imaging [Internet]. 2025; [cited 2025 Jul 10]; Available from: https://pubmed.ncbi.nlm.nih.gov/40531649/
27. Brown M, Schoen JH, Gross J, Omary RA, Hanneman K. Climate change and radiology: impetus for change and a toolkit for action. Radiology [Internet]. 2023;307(4) [cited 2025 Aug 12] https://doi.org/10.1148/radiol.230229.

28. Picano E, Mangia C, D'Andrea A. Climate change, carbon dioxide emissions, and medical imaging contribution. J Clin Med [Internet]. 2023;12(1) [cited 2025 Aug 12]. Available from: https://pubmed.ncbi.nlm.nih.gov/36615016/
29. Woolen SA, Kim CJ, Hernandez AM, Becker A, Martin AJ, Kuoy E, et al. Radiology environmental impact: what is known and how can we improve? Acad Radiol [Internet]. 2023;30(4):625–30. [cited 2025 Aug 12]; Available from: https://www.sciencedirect.com/science/article/pii/S1076633222005773
30. Doo FX, Vosshenrich J, Cook TS, Moy L, Almeida EPRP, Woolen SA, et al. Environmental sustainability and AI in radiology: a double-edged sword. Radiology. Radiological Society of North America Inc. 2024;310
31. Rudie JD, Gleason T, Barkovich MJ, Wilson DM, Shankaranarayanan A, Zhang T, et al. Clinical assessment of deep learning–based super-resolution for 3D volumetric brain MRI. Radiol Artif Intell. 2022;4(2)
32. Bani-Ahmad M, England A, McLaughlin L, Hadi YH, McEntee M. Potential of artificial intelligence for radiation dose reduction in computed tomography —a scoping review. Radiography [Internet]. 2025;31(4):102968. [cited 2025 Aug 12]; Available from: https://www.sciencedirect.com/science/article/pii/S1078817425001129
33. Shahbandegan A, Mago V, Alaref A, van der Pol CB, Savage DW. Developing a machine learning model to predict patient need for computed tomography imaging in the emergency department. PLoS One. 2022;17(12 December)
34. Kjelle E, Andersen ER, Soril LJJ, van Bodegom-Vos L, Hofmann BM. Interventions to reduce low-value imaging—a systematic review of interventions and outcomes. BMC Health Serv Res. 2021;21(1)
35. Rothenberg S, Bame B, Herskovitz E. Prospective evaluation of a machine-learning prediction model for missed Radiology appointments. J Digit Imaging. 2022;35(6):1690–3.
36. Cicek V, Bagci U. AI-powered contrast-free cardiovascular magnetic resonance imaging for myocardial infarction. Front Cardiovasc Med [Internet]. 2024;11:1457498. [cited 2025 Aug 12]; Available from: https://pmc.ncbi.nlm.nih.gov/articles/PMC11617551/
37. Chandrashekar A, Handa A, Lapolla P, Shivakumar N, Uberoi R, Grau V, et al. A deep learning approach to visualize aortic aneurysm morphology without the use of intravenous contrast agents. Ann Surg [Internet]. 2023;277(2):E449–59. [cited 2025 Jul 18]; Available from: https://journals.lww.com/annalsofsurgery/fulltext/2023/02000/a_deep_learning_approach_to_visualize_aortic.54.aspx
38. Dayarathna S, Islam KT, Uribe S, Yang G, Hayat M, Chen Z. Deep learning based synthesis of MRI, CT and PET: review and analysis. Med Image Anal [Internet]. 2024;92:103046. [cited 2025 Aug 12]; Available from: https://www.sciencedirect.com/science/article/pii/S1361841523003067

39. Schwartz R, Dodge J, Smith NA, Etzioni O. Green AI. Commun ACM [Internet]. 2020;63(12):54–63. [cited 2025 Jul 18]; Available from: https://dl.acm.org/doi/pdf/10.1145/3381831
40. Kocak B, Ponsiglione A, Romeo V, Ugga L, Huisman M, Cuocolo R. Radiology AI and sustainability paradox: environmental, economic, and social dimensions. Insights Imaging [Internet]. 2025;16(1):88. [cited 2025 Aug 11]; Available from: https://pmc.ncbi.nlm.nih.gov/articles/PMC12006592/
41. Thangam D, Muniraju H, Ramesh R, Narasimhaiah R, Muddasir N, Khan A, et al. Impact of data centers on power consumption, climate change, and sustainability. 2024. [cited 2025 Aug 12]; Available from: www.irma-international.org/chapter/digital-forensics-in-distributed-environment/224626
42. Anthony LFW, Kanding B, Selvan R. Carbontracker: tracking and predicting the carbon footprint of training deep learning models. 2020. [cited 2025 Jul 18]; Available from: https://arxiv.org/pdf/2007.03051

# 3 Sustainability in Healthcare from the Radiological Perspective

Helena M. Dekker

## 3.1 Introduction

Medical facilities require significant energy to power computing systems, equipment, heating, and cooling. The healthcare sector accounts for 10% of all materials consumed globally each year [1] and contributes 4.5% of total greenhouse gas (GHG) emissions worldwide.

Radiology departments, in particular, are characterized by high energy consumption due to numerous medical devices, extensive use of contrast media, large-scale data storage, and frequent patient logistics. Additionally, they rely on a substantial number of disposable items, including syringes, tubes, needles, biopsy needles, drains, and gloves.

The extensive use of contrast media in radiology warrants serious attention due to its environmental impact, particularly on aquatic ecosystems, and the reliance on finite natural resources for its production. As CT and MRI examinations constitute a crit-

H. M. Dekker (✉)
Department of Medical Imaging, Radboud University Medical Center, Nijmegen, The Netherlands
e-mail: heleen.dekker@radboudumc.nl





E. R. Ranschaert et al. (eds.), *Sustainability of AI in Radiology*, Imaging Informatics for Healthcare Professionals,
https://doi.org/10.1007/978-3-032-15693-8_3

ical component of diagnostic and therapeutic pathways, their utilization must be optimized to minimize associated energy consumption.

Recent advances in artificial intelligence (AI) have begun to demonstrate promising potential in supporting radiologists, particularly in streamlining workflows and enhancing diagnostic efficiency.

To accelerate the transition towards sustainable radiology, institutional policies and the strategic agendas of professional societies must proactively integrate and promote these developments. Addressing the issue of sustainability in radiology requires collaboration with all stakeholders: radiologists, manufacturers, and patients.

## 3.2 Contrast Media

Contrast media are essential for diagnostic and interventional procedures. The rapid increase in the use of medical imaging during the last few decades has resulted in a substantial increase in the use of contrast media. Over the last 20 years, scanner availability has rapidly increased in most countries. Iodinated contrast media (ICM) are the most frequently used, particularly in CT scans. As a result, many millions of litres (estimated more than ten million litres) of ICM are used globally every year [2]. Gadolinium-based contrast agents (GBCA) are only used in small quantities on a per-patient basis; this results in the use of many thousands of litres of GBCA per year (estimated more than half a million litres) [3].

Data show that these ICM and GBCA are present in sewage water, surface water, and drinking water in many regions of the world. Therefore, there is growing concern regarding the environmental impact of ICM and GBCA because of their ubiquitous presence in the aquatic environment [2, 3]. Some iodinated contrast media are susceptible to biotransformation under an/aerobic conditions [4]. During the production of drinking water,

ICM can form iodinated disinfection by-products [5]. Transformation of GBCA can create free gadolinium and lead to the formation of Gd complexes during anaerobic sewage sludge treatment [6].

Addressing the issue of contrast media in water requires collaboration with all stakeholders. Radiologists have a wide spectrum of options to reduce contrast media contrast media (CM) use without compromising diagnostic quality. Manufacturers play a key role by developing more sustainable solutions, optimizing packaging, and facilitating recycling options for leftover CM. Patients can contribute by collecting their urine containing CM, which helps prevent contrast media from entering wastewater systems. There are three potential courses of action to be considered: firstly, optimizing the application of contrast media; secondly, reducing the waste of contrast media; and thirdly, collecting the urine containing excreted contrast media (Table 3.1).

**Table 3.1** Measures to reduce contrast media (CM) and opportunities for implementation

| Measures | Opportunities for implementation |
|---|---|
| To reduce the use of CM | Optimization of protocols<br>Preauthorization of CT and MRI requests<br>Individualizing the volume of contrast media<br>Alternative contrast media |
| To reduce the waste of CM | Multi-patient injection systems and the use of bulk packaging<br>Higher concentration of ICM<br>High-relaxivity GBCA<br>Collection of residues of contrast media<br>Recycling services |
| To reduce the amount of CM excreted into sewage water | Use of urine bags in outpatients<br>Specialized toilet filtration system<br>Prolonged in-hospital time for outpatients |

### 3.2.1 Measures to Reduce the Use of Contrast Agents

#### 3.2.1.1 Optimization of Protocols

Regular updates of CT and MRI protocols are recommended to optimize contrast media use according to the latest scientific insights and the technical capabilities of the scanners in use.

#### 3.2.1.2 Pre-authorization of CT and MRI Requests

Preauthorization of CT and MRI requests by a radiologist provides assessment of the correct indication for these examinations and the correct application of contrast medium. Preauthorization of MRI requests can lead to a significant reduction in the use of these modalities, with a reduction in imaging costs and a reduction in the use of GBCAs [7].

#### 3.2.1.3 Weight-Based Contrast Calculation Volume Reduction

The introduction of individualized intravenous ICM and GBCA volumes, based on the clinical question and personalized to body weight, results in less contrast media being used per patient in most patients.

#### 3.2.1.4 Alternative Contrast Agents

The class of ultra-small superparamagnetic iron oxide particles (USPIOs) may be an alternative to GBCAs with a high safety profile. Their iron content results in a strong T1-relaxation effect, similar to that of GBCAs. The use of USPIO in patients does not pose any known risks to the environment. This is because the USPIO contrast media are metabolized in the patient's body after intravenous administration, and iron is a physiological element that is used in non-toxic concentrations for MR imaging. The iron from the USPIO contrast media is metabolized in the body via the normal iron metabolic cycle, and there is no known excretion of USPIOs as particles after intravenous injection [3].

Manganese-based contrast agents have the potential to replace GBCA, but researchers have yet to address safety adequately [8].

Manganese is a naturally occurring element in the human body and is essential for numerous biological functions, rendering it inherently biocompatible. It is abundantly available from diverse global resources, which are not restricted to a few geographic regions, offering significant potential for the development of sustainable manganese-based contrast agents [9].

### 3.2.2 Measures to Reduce the Waste of Contrast Media

#### 3.2.2.1 Multi-patient Injection Systems and the Use of Bulk Packaging

Multi-patient injection systems allow the use of vial/bottle sizes ranging from 10 ml to 700 ml. This allows the amount of contrast material injected to be individualized without increasing contrast material waste. The system works best by starting the day with a large bottle size and then adjusting the bottle size at the end of the day to the expected total usage for the upcoming scan hours [10], considering the maximum usage time once the bottle stopper has been pierced. This time can vary up to 24 h, depending on the manufacturer. In certain hospitals, internal regulations may limit the use of large-volume bottles. Additionally, the use of a saline flush is crucial for optimal utilization of the contrast medium. Employing larger packaging also contributes to sustainability by reducing overall packaging waste [11].

#### 3.2.2.2 Higher Concentration of Iodinated Contrast Media

Iodinated contrast media are available in various concentrations. A higher iodine concentration allows for a reduction in contrast volume without decreasing the total iodine dose. In other words, the same iodine dose can be delivered using a smaller volume of solution. Using higher concentrations has the added benefit of reducing packaging needs and minimizing residual waste.

Standardizing the use of a high-concentration contrast agent across a department also eliminates the need to switch between different concentrations for different types of examinations, such as cardiac and non-cardiac scans.

#### 3.2.2.3 High-Relaxivity GBCA

Manufacturers have recently developed a new generation of GBCA [9]. These are so-called high-relaxivity macrocyclic contrast agents, whereby the doses to be used can be reduced by half or even more compared to products already available on the market for a longer time. Bracco and Guerbet jointly developed gadopiclenol. FDA and European Medicines Agency (EMA) approvals have been obtained. The brand names are, respectively, Vueway (Bracco Imaging) and Elucirem (Guerbet). Bayer launched gadoquatrane, a tetrameric macrocyclic contrast agent (in late-stage clinical development).

#### 3.2.2.4 Collection of Residues of Contrast Media

Separate collection and disposal of contrast media waste through the hospital's waste management system prevents contrast media from entering the sewerage system. This can be achieved by placing a special container in each CT and MRI suite for the collection of residual contrast media. These containers are disposed of through the hospital's dedicated waste channels and destroyed in an incinerator. In the past, such residues were often disposed of by simply pouring them down the sink.

#### 3.2.2.5 Recycling Services

Contrast media recycling is an emerging practice. Some manufacturers now offer collection and recycling services for uncontaminated leftover contrast media. Special containers are provided to radiology departments and later collected by the manufacturer. The iodine or gadolinium is then extracted from the unused contrast material and reused in industrial applications—effectively extending the material's life cycle.

### 3.2.3 Measures to Reduce the Amount of Contrast Media in Sewage Water

#### 3.2.3.1 Urine Bags After Contrast Administration in Outpatients

In the Netherlands [12, 13] and in Germany [14], pilot studies were performed on outpatients after a contrast-enhanced CT scan. This method could also be used for outpatients after a contrast-enhanced MRI scan, but no such studies of this are known to date. Disposable urine bags contain an absorbent material that holds the urine in place and can be sealed. Patients use the bags at home during the first four urination sessions after the administration of intravenous contrast media. The bags are disposed of via the household waste system. If this domestic waste is further processed in an incinerator, the contrast agent is reduced to naturally occurring iodine and iodine salts [15], which are not known to have a negative environmental impact.

#### 3.2.3.2 Specialized Toilet Filtration System

A specialized toilet filtration system consisting of a separation toilet, urinal, and cartridges is developed. The cartridges contain absorbents that bind contrast media. This system has recently been introduced by a company (Zereau) in the Netherlands. This toilet system can be installed in a hospital radiology department, and patients can use this toilet for their first urination session after contrast-enhanced CT and contrast-enhanced MRI examinations. Initial studies show that the cartridge removal efficiency was close to 100%. The option to filter out contrast agents directly at the source represents a crucial initial step in the recycling process [16].

#### 3.2.3.3 Prolonged In-Hospital Time for Outpatients

In Italy, the Greenwater study was conducted, in which outpatients were asked to stay 1 h longer in hospital after a scheduled contrast-enhanced CT or MRI examination and asked to urinate into a dedicated canister. The median time interval between contrast administration and urine collection was 25 min (ICM) and

24 min (GBCA). The median recovery rate was 51.2% for ICM and 12.9% for GBCA [17]. Patients were willing to stay an extra half-hour after their scans to have their urine collected.

## 3.3 Optimization of Protocols

It is recommended that CT and MRI protocols be updated on a regular basis. Optimization of CT protocols including for radiation exposure (the ALARA principle) and ICM use. Optimization of MRI protocols for new MRI sequences, post-processing, deep learning methods, and the application of abbreviated MRI protocols for specific indications. A reduction in the number of series acquired during CT and MRI examinations leads to shorter scanning times and, consequently, a decrease in unnecessary energy consumption. The advent of improved technology has resulted in a reduction in the necessity for contrast media, or even the complete elimination of such contrast media in certain instances [3, 18]. According to the literature, follow-up of vestibular schwannomas and meningiomas can be performed without contrast media [19, 20].

Postprocessing using artificial intelligence techniques can create 'virtual' or 'augmented' contrast images. Augmented contrast images boost existing contrast enhancement, while virtual post-contrast images use the information available on other sequences of the scan to estimate contrast enhancement [21]. The creation of augmented contrast images is still in the research phase. A related example is the generation of contrast-enhanced CT images within the framework of the NetZeroAICT project [22].

## 3.4 Hardware

A life cycle assessment of a diagnostic radiology department's environmental footprint found that energy consumption from imaging equipment accounts for over 50% of its greenhouse gas (GHG) emissions. MRI is the largest contributor, followed by

CT [1]. For CT, the majority of energy consumption—around two-thirds—occurred during the system's non-productive idle state, indicating low utilization and poor energy efficiency. In this idle state, energy is still consumed to maintain system readiness and to power the cooling systems [23].

To reduce this impact, it is essential to minimize the time imaging equipment spends in unnecessarily high-power modes—for example, remaining in 'ready to scan' mode when low-power mode would suffice, or in low-power mode when it could be turned off entirely. Equipment should be powered down whenever it is not in use.

At the same time, more energy-efficient machines and MRI scanners that use less helium are becoming available. Another promising development is the refurbishment of medical equipment, which requires significantly fewer new raw materials and can have a major environmental benefit.

Modular equipment design, where only a single component needs to be replaced, leads to substantial material savings. Regular maintenance and timely upgrades also help to maximize the equipment's efficiency and lifespan.

## 3.5 Operational Efficiency

An optimized workflow is essential for maximizing scanner efficiency. In practice, this means a high throughput, with examinations scheduled back-to-back, minimizing the time required per patient and reducing scanner idle time. The following factors play an important role in operational efficiency:

- Selecting the appropriate diagnostic examination and getting it right first time
- Minimizing no-shows for outpatient appointments
- Reducing inpatient delays by improving communication with patient transport staff
- Preventing duplicate imaging within a short timeframe
- Optimizing CT and MRI protocols

- Utilizing modern injector systems to streamline radiographer operations and save time
- Optimizing scheduling and increasing patient throughput
- Continue regular maintenance, repairs, and upgrades
- Powering down equipment when not in use (outside regular operating hours)

## 3.6 Artificial Intelligence

While AI tools demonstrate promise in specific clinical areas—such as breast cancer screening—their integration into radiology workflows often introduces additional complexity without robust evidence of improved efficiency or cost-effectiveness [24]. Most existing solutions focus on detection and quantification but still rely heavily on the radiologist's oversight, which limits their practical impact.

To ensure meaningful adoption, there is a clear need for established frameworks that evaluate an AI tool's clinical value, cost-effectiveness, societal impact, explainability, and robustness early in the development process [25].

For effective implementation, domain-specific guidelines, well-defined implementation strategies, and collaborative engagement with all stakeholders—including healthcare professionals, regulators, and industry—are essential [26].

AI is playing an increasingly important role in MRI scans, improving imaging quality and optimizing workflow efficiency. Here are some key applications:

1. Faster Image Acquisition (Accelerated MRI Scans)
   AI algorithms, such as deep learning-based reconstruction techniques (e.g. deep learning MRI reconstruction, as used in DeepResolve by Siemens or AIR Recon DL by GE HealthCare), can significantly reduce scan times.

   This helps lower the energy consumption of MRI scanners and improves patient throughput.

2. Automatic Segmentation and Detection of Abnormalities
   AI models can automatically segment anatomical structures and detect pathologies, such as brain structures in neurodegenerative diseases or tumours in oncological imaging. This could potentially result in a reduced reading time over the longer term.
3. Radiomics and Predictive Models
   AI can transform MRI images into quantitative biomarkers (radiomics), which are valuable for personalized medicine.

   Machine learning models assist in the early detection of diseases, such as Alzheimer's disease or prostate cancer. This could potentially result in a reduced reading time, in combination with improved diagnostic accuracy.

AI is increasingly being used in CT scans to improve image quality, reduce radiation dose, and optimize workflow efficiency. Here are some key applications:

1. Dose Reduction (Lower Radiation Levels While Maintaining Image Quality)
   AI-based image reconstruction algorithms (such as Deep Learning Image Reconstruction (DLIR) by GE or Precise Image by Canon) enable the acquisition of high-quality images with reduced radiation exposure and thus reduced energy consumption.
2. Image Enhancement and Artefact Reduction
   AI helps reduce noise and correct motion artefacts, particularly in patients who struggle to remain still (e.g. children or ICU patients). This avoids the need for repeated scans, thereby reducing energy consumption.

   Deep learning-driven reconstruction can also enhance contrast resolution, allowing for lower doses of contrast agents.
3. Automated Detection and Characterization of Abnormalities
   AI models can automatically identify and categorize lung nodules, fractures, vascular stenosis, and other pathologies. This accelarates diagnosis and assists radiologists in prioritizing critical findings, such as lung cancer or pulmonary embolisms in emergency cases.

4. Radiomics and Quantitative Image Analysis
   AI can extract subtle biomarkers from CT images, supporting personalized medicine and prognosis predictions (e.g. tumour response in oncology).
   AI-powered perfusion analysis is used in stroke imaging to quickly determine which brain regions are salvageable.

## 3.7 Awareness and Active Anticipation Among Radiologists

Creating awareness is essential. As healthcare professionals, we are trained to prioritize patient care. For radiologists, image quality is paramount, and the use of contrast media is often necessary to answer clinical questions. Naturally, we prefer high-quality images and plenty of them. However, many radiologists have not given much thought to the consumption of resources, equipment, energy, and the environmental impact of our practice.

As healthcare professionals, we also have a responsibility for environmental sustainability. In our daily work, we should remain mindful of our ecological footprint. Awareness of our environmental impact must be followed by active participation in initiatives aimed at reducing resource consumption, including energy use and contrast media.

## 3.8 Green Team

Successful implementation of sustainability in radiology requires a dedicated approach within the department. An imaging sustainability group or committee (green team) is essential to drive and integrate sustainable practices effectively. This team, with a diverse representation of staff roles to reflect the operations of the department, should consist of at least radiologists, radiographers, policy officers, clinical scientists, and managers/administrators.

At the Department of Medical Imaging at Radboud University Medical Center, a green team was established, consisting of staff members from various professional roles. This multidisciplinary approach fosters meaningful interaction and valuable contributions from the workplace.

The green team plays a crucial role in initiating and overseeing sustainability initiatives, ensuring that environmental considerations become an integral part of daily radiology practice. By working together, these professionals may also undertake audit, training, research and other related activities. There is a reporting system in place to publicize the work of the group and increase awareness of sustainability.

## 3.9 Radiological Societies

At a national level, each radiological society can take responsibility by establishing a dedicated working group or committee for sustainability. This committee can define clear sustainability goals and communicate them to all members, ensuring a coordinated effort towards greener radiology practices. The radiological society can also promote sustainability education by integrating this topic into training courses for residents. Furthermore, sustainability can be incorporated into quality assurance visits.

A supporting website could serve as a valuable resource, offering tips and best practices for integrating sustainability into daily radiology workflows. Additionally, sustainability should become a recurring topic on the agenda of national radiology conferences, fostering awareness and knowledge-sharing among professionals.

Collaboration with the national society of radiographers is also key, as both professions play a crucial role in implementing sustainable practices. Furthermore, the national committee can conduct surveys to monitor the progress of sustainability integration across hospitals, helping to identify challenges and share successful strategies.

By taking these steps, radiological societies can lead the way in embedding sustainability into clinical practice and healthcare policy.

## 3.10 European Initiatives for Sustainable Radiology

At the European level, the European Society of Radiology (ESR) has established a Subcommittee on Sustainability. This subcommittee focuses on awareness, education, and the integration of sustainability into radiology practice.

One of its key initiatives is the development of a GreenID certification for radiology departments, which aims to set sustainability standards and encourage environmentally responsible practices. While this project is still in its early stages, it represents a significant step towards greener radiology.

During ESR 2025, sustainability was a key topic, and the subcommittee played an important role in shaping discussions and initiatives. Moving forward, the subcommittee will continue to drive efforts to embed sustainability into radiology at a European level, ensuring long-term impact across the field.

The MeGadoRe Project (*Medical Gadolinium Recycling*) is a French initiative focused on the recycling of gadolinium. Based at the Faculty of Science and Technology in Brest, the project aims to reduce the ecological footprint of medical procedures by recovering and reusing gadolinium.

The MeGadoRe team consists of experts working together to develop innovative methods for efficiently recycling gadolinium. Through these efforts, the project seeks to minimize the environmental impact of contrast agents while decreasing reliance on newly extracted gadolinium.

For more information about the MeGadoRe Project and its research, visit its official website: megadore.org.

## 3.11 Changes in Working Practice

Within radiology, there is still a great deal of potential for savings through the introduction of the measures mentioned. With the introduction of improved CT and MRI protocols, significant results can be achieved quickly by reducing the use of contrast agents. This also applies to creating a more efficient workflow in CT and MRI, leading to lower energy consumption. As a result, this immediately contributes to cost reduction within a radiology department.

Conduct regular small-scale audits within your department—for example, check whether equipment is turned off outside office hours. And if devices must remain on, ensure they are set to the lowest possible energy mode.

Consider investing in software and AI solutions that support more efficient workflows while also taking their energy consumption into account.

If we can take the next step of recycling a portion of the contrast agents from patients' urine, we will reduce the need for raw materials. Iodine and gadolinium are mined resources that are in high demand and becoming increasingly scarce.

Collaboration with all stakeholders is crucial for the development of new sustainability initiatives.

Optimizing the entire patient process—the patient journey—within radiology and across our hospitals is essential. This means that a hospital-wide vision regarding sustainability needs to be established too. At the same time, improving the development, production, and use of all devices and materials involved will contribute to more sustainable and efficient healthcare delivery.

To take further steps, awareness, education, scientific research, and collaboration between all stakeholders are essential to reduce the ecological footprint of radiology.

With this chapter, I hope to deliver a wake-up call and thereby contribute to the sustainability of radiology departments.

## References

1. Thiel CL, Vigil-Garcia M, Nande S, Meijer C, Gehrels J, Struk O, Thornander S, Pullella D, Omary RA, Carver DE, Scheel JR. Environmental life cycle assessment of a U.S. hospital-based radiology practice. Radiology. 2024;313(2):e240398. https://doi.org/10.1148/radiol.240398. PMID: 39589247; PMCID: PMC11605107
2. Dekker HM, Stroomberg GJ, Prokop M. Tackling the increasing contamination of the water supply by iodinated contrast media. Insights Imaging.

2022;13(1):30. https://doi.org/10.1186/s13244-022-01175-x. PMID: 35201493; PMCID: PMC8873335

3. Dekker HM, Stroomberg GJ, Van der Molen AJ, Prokop M. Review of strategies to reduce the contamination of the water environment by gadolinium-based contrast agents. Insights Imaging. 2024;15(1):62. https://doi.org/10.1186/s13244-024-01626-7. PMID: 38411847; PMCID: PMC10899148
4. Redeker M, Wick A, Meermann B, Ternes TA. Anaerobic transformation of the iodinated X-ray contrast medium iopromide, its aerobic transformation products, and transfer to further iodinated X-ray contrast media. Environ Sci Technol. 2018;52(15):8309–20. https://doi.org/10.1021/acs.est.8b01140. Epub 2018 Jul 12. PMID: 29998733
5. Duirk SE, Lindell C, Cornelison CC, Kormos J, Ternes TA, Attene-Ramos M, Osiol J, Wagner ED, Plewa MJ, Richardson SD. Formation of toxic iodinated disinfection by-products from compounds used in medical imaging. Environ Sci Technol. 2011;45(16):6845–54. https://doi.org/10.1021/es200983f. Epub 2011 Jul 15. PMID: 21761849
6. Telgmann L, Wehe CA, Birka M, Künnemeyer J, Nowak S, Sperling M, Karst U. Speciation and isotope dilution analysis of gadolinium-based contrast agents in wastewater. Environ Sci Technol. 2012;46(21):11929–36. https://doi.org/10.1021/es301981z. Epub 2012 Oct 26. PMID: 23062026
7. Blachar A, Tal S, Mandel A, et al. Preauthorisation of CT and MRI examinations: assessment of a managed care Preauthorisation program based on the ACR appropriateness criteria and the Royal College of Radiology guidelines. J Am Coll Radiol. 2006;3:851–9.
8. Davis KA, Lazar B. Manganese-based contrast agents as a replacement for gadolinium. Radiol Technol. 2021;93(1):36–45. PMID: 34588277
9. Frenzel T, Wels T, Pietsch H, Schöckel L, Seidensticker P, Endrikat J. Recent developments and future perspectives in magnetic resonance imaging and computed tomography contrast media. Invest Radiol. 2025; https://doi.org/10.1097/RLI.0000000000001180. Epub ahead of print. PMID: 40163898
10. Struik F, Futterer JJ, Prokop WM. Performance of single-use syringe versus multi-use MR contrast injectors: a prospective comparative study. Sci Rep. 2020;10(1):3946. https://doi.org/10.1038/s41598-020-60697-w. PMID: 32127584; PMCID: PMC7054519
11. Lindsey JS, Frederick-Dyer K, Carr JJ, Cooke E, Allen LM, Omary RA. Modeling the environmental and financial impact of multi-dose vs. single-dose iodinated contrast media packaging and delivery systems. Acad Radiol. 2023;30(6):1017–23. https://doi.org/10.1016/j.acra.2022.12.029. Epub 2023 Jan 6. PMID: 36621442
12. Hoogenboom J, Bergema K, van Vliet BJM, Hendriksen A. Eindrapportage Brede Plaszakkenproef. 2021

13. Dekker HM, Beltman HB, Prokop M. Are patients willing to help reduce contrast material in the environment? The outpatient use of urine bags after contrast-enhanced computed tomography. Eur Radiol. 2025; https://doi.org/10.1007/s00330-025-11565-6. Epub ahead of print. PMID: 40216613
14. Röntgenkrontrastmittel in der Ruhr: Pilotproject. www.merkmal-ruhr.de
15. Ooms J, Steketee J, Kupfernagel J. Milieu-impactstudie afvoeren contrastmiddelen via riool of plaszak. Report number: R001-1244410JUO-bebV01-NL. 2016;
16. Dekker HM, Talsma A, Hol A, Prokop M. Reducing the amount of excreted contrast media in sewage water: a pilot study using a specialized toilet filter system. RSNA. 2024;
17. Zanardo M, Ambrogi F, Asmundo L, Cardani R, Cirillo G, Colarieti A, Cozzi A, Cressoni M, Dambra I, Di Leo G, Monti CB, Nicotera L, Pomati F, Renna LV, Secchi F, Versuraro M, Vitali P, Sardanelli F. The GREENWATER study: patients' green sensitivity and potential recovery of injected contrast agents. Eur Radiol. 2025;35(3):1205–14. https://doi.org/10.1007/s00330-024-11150-3. Epub 2024 Oct 31. PMID: 39480535
18. Tsui B, Calabrese E, Zaharchuk G, Rauschecker AM. Reducing gadolinium contrast with Artificial Intelligence. J Magn Reson Imaging. 2024;60(3):848–59. https://doi.org/10.1002/jmri.29095. Epub 2023 Oct 31. PMID: 37905681
19. Kim DH, Lee S, Hwang SH. Non-contrast magnetic resonance imaging for diagnosis and monitoring of vestibular Schwannomas: a systematic review and meta-analysis. Otol Neurotol. 2019;40(9):1126–33. https://doi.org/10.1097/MAO.0000000000002416. PMID: 31469788
20. Rahatli FK, Donmez FY, Kesim C, Haberal KM, Turnaoglu H, Agildere AM. Can unenhanced brain magnetic resonance imaging be used in routine follow up of meningiomas to avoid gadolinium deposition in brain? Clin Imaging. 2019;53:155–61. https://doi.org/10.1016/j.clinimag.2018.10.014. Epub 2018 Oct 13. PMID: 30343167
21. Pasquini L, Napolitano A, Pignatelli M, Tagliente E, Parrillo C, Nasta F, Romano A, Bozzao A, Di Napoli A. Synthetic post-contrast imaging through Artificial Intelligence: clinical applications of virtual and augmented contrast media. Pharmaceutics. 2022;14(11):2378. https://doi.org/10.3390/pharmaceutics14112378.
22. Chandrashekar A, Shivakumar N, Lapolla P, Handa A, Grau V, Lee R. Oxford Abdominal Aortic Aneurysm (OxAAA) Study, A deep learning approach to generate contrast-enhanced computerised tomography angiograms without the use of intravenous contrast agents. European Heart Journal. 2020;41(Suppl 2):ehaa946.0156. https://doi.org/10.1093/ehjci/ehaa946.0156.

23. Heye T, Knoerl R, Wehrle T, Mangold D, Cerminara A, Loser M, Plumeyer M, Degen M, Lüthy R, Brodbeck D, Merkle E. The energy consumption of radiology: energy- and cost-saving opportunities for CT and MRI operation. Radiology. 2020;295(3):593–605. https://doi.org/10.1148/radiol.2020192084. Epub 2020 Mar 24. PMID: 32208096
24. Huisman M, van Ginneken B, Harvey H. The emperor has few clothes: a realistic appraisal of current AI in radiology. Eur Radiol. 2024;34(9):5873–5. https://doi.org/10.1007/s00330-024-10664-0. Epub 2024 Mar 7. PMID: 38451323
25. Kemper EHM, Erenstein H, Boverhof BJ, Redekop K, Andreychenko AE, Dietzel M, Groot Lipman KBW, Huisman M, Klontzas ME, Vos F, IJzerman M, MPA S, Visser JJ. ESR Essentials: how to get to valuable radiology AI: the role of early health technology assessment-practice recommendations by the European Society of Medical Imaging Informatics. Eur Radiol. 2024; https://doi.org/10.1007/s00330-024-11188-3. Epub ahead of print. PMID: 39636421
26. Kotter E, D'Antonoli TA, Cuocolo R, Hierath M, Huisman M, Klontzas ME, Martí-Bonmatí L, May MS, Neri E, Nikolaou K, Pinto Dos Santos D, Radzina M, Shelmerdine SC, Bellemo A. European Society of Radiology (ESR). Guiding AI in radiology: ESR's recommendations for effective implementation of the European AI Act. Insights Imaging. 2025;16(1):33. https://doi.org/10.1186/s13244-025-01905-x. PMID: 39948192; PMCID: PMC11825415

# 4 Environmental Footprint of Radiology and the Role of AI in Obtaining Sustainability for Radiology

Neil Lall, Douglas Spaeth-Cook, and Nabile Safdar

## 4.1 Introduction

Despite its crucial role in modern healthcare, radiology unfortunately contributes significantly to the healthcare sector's environmental footprint, primarily through the manufacturing and energy-intensive use of imaging equipment [1, 2]. Emitting more than 2 gigatons of $CO_2$ equivalent annually, the healthcare sector accounts for approximately 5–10% of greenhouse gas emissions in developed nations. In the United States, this amounts to ~8.5% (~546 $MtCO_2e$), while in the European Union, it represents ~4.7% (~249 $MtCO_2e$). Most of these emissions arise from supply chains (Scope 3, ~75%), with smaller contributions from direct emissions (Scope 1, ~14%), and purchased energy (Scope 2, ~11%)

N. Lall (✉) · N. Safdar
Department of Radiology, Emory University, Children's Healthcare of Atlanta, Atlanta, GA, USA
e-mail: neil.uttam.lall@emory.edu; nabile.m.safdar@emory.edu

D. Spaeth-Cook
Department of Radiology, Emory University, Atlanta, GA, USA
e-mail: douglas.spaeth-cook@emory.edu



E. R. Ranschaert et al. (eds.), *Sustainability of AI in Radiology*, Imaging Informatics for Healthcare Professionals,
https://doi.org/10.1007/978-3-032-15693-8_4

[3]. Medical imaging alone is estimated to contribute up to 1% of global greenhouse gas emissions [4, 5]. From 2003 to 2013, these greenhouse gas emissions from the healthcare sector increased by roughly 30% [6]. Growing use of AI and other technological advances in radiology will likely further increase the data storage and computational energy requirements of the field [2, 7].

However, radiology can, and arguably should, also leverage efficiency gains that AI could offer to achieve a net reduction in the field's emissions. As radiology departments strive to balance operational needs with sustainability, AI has emerged as both a challenge and a potential solution. This chapter explores the environmental impact of radiology and examines how AI can help mitigate this footprint while enhancing healthcare delivery.

## 4.2 Energy Consumption in Radiology

### 4.2.1 Types of Radiological Equipment and Energy Expenditure

Medical imaging devices such as computed tomography (CT), magnetic resonance imaging (MRI), ultrasound, and X-ray systems consume substantial energy in both their production and use. The estimated energy emissions involved in manufacturing a single MRI machine are 792,100 kg $CO_2$ equivalent, compared to 697,500 kg for a CT machine and 61,576 kg for an ultrasound machine [8]. For image acquisition, MRI is also the most energy intensive, requiring continuous operation of superconducting magnets and extensive cooling systems for operation, producing an estimated 13,72 kg $CO_2$ equivalent per exam. CT requires high-powered X-ray tubes and rapid image acquisition but uses considerably less energy for image acquisition, emitting an estimated 2,61 kg $CO_2$ equivalent per scan. For image production, ultrasound has the lowest footprint of the three, with an estimated 0,65 kg $CO_2$ equivalent created per exam. Studies evaluating the annual power expenditure of different modalities have found fluoroscopy systems to use approximately three times the energy of ultrasound machines and one third of CT during their analysis [9].

Beyond emissions related to production and use, these systems also have significant emissions that occur during "nonproductive" periods. A systematic review of 11 studies on energy efficiency in radiology found that 40–91% of energy consumed by radiological devices occurs in these nonproductive periods, primarily during idle periods when machines remain powered on but unused [10].

To allow for transparency and informed sustainable purchasing decisions, the US Environmental Protection Agency has recently developed a new Energy Star product specification for medical imaging equipment [11]. As of now, no European body offers a dedicated ecolabel or energy-efficiency certification for medical imaging equipment comparable to the US ENERGY STAR program. Europe relies on broader eco-design standards (e.g., IEC 60601-1-9) or voluntary labels that do not extend to clinical imaging modalities.

### 4.2.2 PC Energy Expenditure for Routine Radiology Uses

In addition to imaging equipment, radiology departments rely heavily on computer workstations for image processing, storage, and interpretation. Picture Archiving and Communication Systems (PACS) and Radiology Information Systems (RIS) run on high-performance computers that operate continuously, adding to the department's energy demands. The norm in many practices in the United States is for the radiology workstations to remain turned on every hour of every day. Estimates for yearly energy expenditure of devices left on 24/7 can be up to 2358.72 kWh for a radiology workstation and 1399.84 kWh for a radiology monitor, though turning them off after work hours and on weekends can reduce this impact by over 75% [12].

### 4.2.3 Imaging Data Storage: On-Premises vs. Cloud-Based

Radiology generates vast amounts of imaging data, necessitating efficient storage solutions. Although cloud computing data centers are now responsible for approximately 1.5% of global energy consumption [13, 14], moving data to the cloud can often reduce the carbon footprint of an organization. Some of the key variables in determining a data center's footprint are server utilization, power usage efficiency, hardware efficiency, and carbon emissions of the electric supply. Server utilization is often optimized by cloud servers due to their economies of scale, while the latter two factors are more likely, but not guaranteed, to be optimized in a cloud environment. However, these are not guarantees, and the "greenness" of the electric supply of different servers in different locations can vary drastically. Because of this, the potential emissions of an on-premises server and a cloud server can significantly overlap.

### 4.2.4 Energy Expenditure for AI

With AI-driven applications gaining traction in radiology, computational power requirements have surged. Training AI models, especially deep learning and generative AI models, is energy-intensive. The training phase of a large language model (LLM) can consume thousands of megawatt-hours (MWh) and generate hundreds of tons of $CO_2$ emissions from running graphics processing units (GPUs) or tensor processing units (TPUs) for weeks or months. Training GPT-3 (175B parameters) required 1287 MWh (equal to approximately 120 US homes' yearly consumption) and is estimated to have emitted 552 tons of $CO_2$ [15]. Newer models such as GPT-4 are speculated to have required 10 to 50 times as much energy, although OpenAI has not disclosed the actual training energy use or $CO_2$ emissions (per Stanford's Foundation Model Transparency Index, which notes that GPT-4's energy data remains undisclosed) [16].

Inference, or the actual use of the trained models, has much lower energy expenditure associated with it, estimated to be near 0.0003 kWh for GPT-3 [17]. While the training phase uses far more energy than a single inference, the inferences for popular LLMs may be run millions of times a day, quickly adding up to surpass the training emissions.

However, as we write this in early 2025, the recent releases of LLMs by DeepSeek and Baidu have highlighted that advances in improving such efficiency can be achieved. Specifically, DeepSeek V3's training required approximately ten times less compute than Meta's similarly performing LLaMa 3.1405B [18]. Baidu's new arrivals claim even more impressive efficiency gains, with the ERNIE X1 LLM reportedly requiring 50% of the expenditures of DeepSeek's more energy-efficient R1 model and ERNIE 4.5 requiring only 1% of OpenAI's GPT-4.5 [19].

Additionally, it is important to note that the data centers upon which AI operations rely are the source of many of these greenhouse gas emissions due to electricity consumption. As discussed above, there can be significant variations in the carbon footprints of data centers. In addition to the electric supply and heating/cooling considerations weighing in to the overall data center footprint, when used for AI models, use of specifically tuned accelerators in the data centers can also achieve up to five times the efficiency of off-the-shelf systems [15].

## 4.3 The Role of AI in Achieving Sustainability in Radiology

While the primary goal of medicine is to save lives and enhance well-being, the environmental impact of our practices can inadvertently cause long-term harm to the very patients we aim to protect. Radiology is one of the most energy-intensive aspects of medicine, contributing significantly to the carbon footprint of healthcare facilities. As discussed, the data and computational needs of AI have the potential to significantly increase this carbon footprint. As such, it is vital to take into consideration ways in which AI usage in radiology may mitigate this capacity for environmental damage.

### 4.3.1 Schedule Optimization

AI can streamline radiology workflows, reducing unnecessary imaging, optimizing scanner usage, and improving reporting efficiency. Automated scheduling and protocol selection help minimize machine idle time and energy waste.

AI tools able to optimize operational efficiency could reduce emissions through decreasing idle time in the imaging workflow. Predictive models could accomplish this through multiple means, such as setting staffing levels based on anticipated workload or dynamically adjusting the patient exam schedule to fit the needs of each specific study. The latter is perhaps best illustrated with MRI. Rather than having MRI time slots determined based on a few simple criteria (such as the general exam type ordered and the need for sedation), these could be dynamically adjusted using parameters such as the specific MRI sequences protocoled, patient size, and scan time for that patient's prior exams. Additional methods for increasing schedule efficiency could include processes to simplify and expedite the technologist workflow like AI-driven automation of exam planning/documentation steps. Examples of this could include automated imaging plane selection for MRI and automated exam labeling for ultrasound [1].

These and other similar operational optimizations would allow condensing the preexisting workload into a smaller operational window, which would have the benefit of decreasing both costs and emissions and increasing productivity. Resultant decreased staffing needs would decrease indirect emissions related to staff commutes. However, larger reductions in emissions can come from minimizing the time imaging equipment spends in unproductive "idle" states, which still consume a moderate degree of energy. One study found that switching MRI scanners from idle to off overnight reduced energy use by 25–33% annually, while employing a "power-save" mode yielded a total reduction of 46–51% compared to idle [20]. Most current implementations rely on manual protocols or scheduler-driven shutdowns, although some vendors now offer power-save software features. For more on these emerging capabilities, see the *Power Management* section (4.3.2). Schedule optimization would ensure the machines spend more time in their productive state of image acquisition and are able to enter low-energy consumption "off" or "standby" states when not used. One analysis of MRI energy use found that increasing scanner utilization from 30% to 90% yielded a nearly threefold reduction in per-patient energy consumption, primarily by spreading the scanner's fixed baseline energy demand across more patients rather than reducing the absolute daily energy use [21]. In the long run, increasing the patient throughput per modality unit would also decrease the need for additional units, with associated decreases in production-related emissions of those additional units.

Additional methods to improve operational efficiency while reducing costs could involve greater enabling of same-day exam scheduling for patients, streamlining the patients' schedules to consolidate appointments into a single visit, and matching patients to shorter commutes to get their needed imaging. All of these would decrease miles driven, thus reducing emissions related to our field.

| Workflow step | Example AI intervention | Mechanism of emission reduction |
|---|---|---|
| Exam scheduling and protocoling | Dynamic slot allocation for MRI, automated protocol selection | Reduces idle scanner time, enables standby modes |
| Staffing | Predictive workload modeling | Decreases unnecessary staffing, reduces commute-related emissions |
| Technologist workflow | Automated plane selection (MRI), auto-labeling (ultrasound) | Increases throughput, reduces equipment idle time |
| Patient scheduling | Same-day scheduling, consolidated appointments | Decreases repeat trips to hospital, reduces patient travel emissions |
| Patient-site matching | Assigning patients to closest imaging center | Shorter commutes → less transport-related $CO_2$ |
| Equipment life cycle | Higher throughput per scanner | Decreases need for additional scanner production |

### 4.3.2 Power Management

One straightforward method to temper the energy-intensive nature of imaging equipment would be to reduce the time these systems spend in their nonproductive states. Predictive AI models could play an important role in this realm by monitoring imaging workflow patterns and autonomously switching systems to lower-energy standby or "off" modes. Even simple, non-AI-related energy-saving strategies have been shown to have the potential for up to 171,000 kWh of savings per device per year [10].

Though a smaller overall contributor, radiology workstations also have potential energy savings of up to 75% if turned off outside of work hours [12, 22]. Expert commentary has similarly emphasized practical strategies such as shortening standby delays (e.g., from 4 h to 1 h, achieving a 45% reduction in idle consumption), implementing energy-monitoring dashboards, and developing workflow-aligned shutdown protocols [23]. While these actions may not fundamentally require an AI model, dynamic scheduling could be highly beneficial; decreased radiologist productivity from waiting for radiology workstations to boot from the off state has been calculated to be more than double the cost of the electricity saved by turning off workstations [24]. Given the shift work inherent to radiology as well as software updates that may need to occur during off hours, usage hours can vary significantly from workstation to workstation and from day to day. The same concepts of dynamically adjusting the hardware power state based upon predicted usage needs could be applied to workstations to achieve additional power savings. This idea could also be expanded to reduce many different sources of energy expenditure in radiology departments, such as dynamic adjustment of light, ventilation, or temperature [25]. The latter is an especially important consideration given the major contributions to emissions from climate control, particularly in interventional radiology.

### 4.3.3 Optimization of Data Management

Data storage is a relatively small component of radiology's overall emissions, though it is likely to grow as data volumes continue to increase. While the footprint of cloud storage can vary drastically, it in general is more energy efficient than on-premises storage. However, some of the considerations at play in determining such energy needs are server utilization, power usage efficiency, hardware efficiency, climate control needs, and the "greenness" of its electric supply. Additionally, different types of storage media provide differing footprints; for example, tape requires relatively little power but is not appropriate for rapid access to data.

AI models that can predict the need for specific data can optimize its distribution between rapid-access on-premises, edge servers, and more remote energy-efficient cloud servers. Similarly, such models could optimize the physical medium for specific data based on its space, access speed, and energy usage. Intelligent pre-fetching of necessary data would allow rapid access to needed data while ensuring low-urgency data is stored as efficiently as possible. Additionally, such optimization of data availability would reduce the frequency of unnecessary data transfers, a process that also consumes additional energy.

### 4.3.4 Extend Hardware Capabilities

Emissions related to the production and transport of goods and services (also known as Scope 3 indirect emissions) comprise a large portion of radiology's ecological footprint [21]. As such, it is vital that our efforts to decrease emissions also target our supply chain.

As AI models are developed to expand our diagnostic capabilities, an important area of focus will be the use of software to improve the quality of imaging from aging equipment in ways that can make it more comparable to imaging from newer devices.

Such developments could prolong the life of older hardware if software enhancements are able to produce equivalent state-of-the-art images.

The same advances can be employed to allow newer hardware to be fundamentally more power-efficient. For example, AI-based augmentation of images from low-field-strength (< 1 T) and ultra-low-field-strength (< 0.1 T) MRI systems could allow these to achieve greater adoption in clinical practice. These low-field-strength systems can significantly reduce energy use in both the production and use phases [1].

### 4.3.5 Reducing Energy Expenditure in Image Acquisition

AI-based image processing and synthesis could also be a path to decreased emissions. For example, AI-based image acquisition acceleration algorithms could allow for lower radiation dose in CT, thereby decreasing the overall energy expenditure of exam acquisition. Such algorithms have even more potential for energy savings during MRI, which is a very time-consuming and energy-intensive examination. With a linear correlation between the length and emissions related to an individual MRI sequence, accelerating acquisition of these sequences can allow for significant decreases in direct energy expenditure, particularly as acceleration factors of up to 100x are being explored [1].

Moreover, shortening examinations could also allow for significant downstream emission reductions. Given the long length of MRIs, sedation is a common necessity for such examinations, particularly in pediatric populations. Sedation not only requires the use of additional materials (often resulting in disposable waste) and additional electricity to power its equipment but also involves significant environmental release of anesthetic gases. These gases have up to 1000 times the global warming effects of carbon dioxide, and unfortunately, 80–95% of the gases administered are vented into the atmosphere rather than being metabolized by the patients [26].

### 4.3.6 Reducing Use of Contrast Agents and Radioisotopes

AI tools also have the potential to decrease the use of intravenous contrast through several means. This could range from algorithms that can increase the conspicuity of decreased contrast doses or could even potentially obviate the need for contrast altogether with optimized virtual calculated post-contrast images from non-contrast examinations [27]. A particularly promising example is the *NetZeroAICT* project, an EU-funded initiative developing AI-driven "digital contrast" technology that synthesizes contrast-enhanced images from non-contrast CTs, offering an eco-friendly, cost-effective, and patient-safer alternative to iodinated contrast media [28]. AI assistance could also be beneficial in the research and development of the contrast agents themselves, by helping with the molecular design of higher-relaxivity contrast agents that will allow for usage of smaller doses of contrast medium. Reducing dependence on contrast agents will allow a decreased footprint in the mining of rare earth metals as well as in aspects like decreased product packaging and transportation. Additionally, our decreased use of contrast media will decrease the downstream accumulation in water supplies.

Radioisotopes are expensive and resource-intensive to make and transport, and they can carry associated radiation risks for patients and family members. Similar AI models could be used to reduce the dose of radioisotopes needed for certain examinations, with similar augmentation of the signal obtained from a smaller dose.

### 4.3.7 Clinical Decision Support

Clinical decision support (CDS) systems provide real-time guidance to clinicians at the point of care to help inform decisions about a patient's care. For example, the American College of Radiology (ACR) has developed Appropriateness Criteria that are used in CDS tools to assist in determining the optimal imaging studies for different scenarios. These systems can prompt clinicians to reconsider or modify orders that do not meet established guidelines, thereby reducing the number of inappropriate or low-utility imaging studies. Existing systems without AI assistance have been found to decrease inappropriate orders by up to 26% [29]. Additionally, because these systems can expedite scheduling of exams rather than awaiting prior authorization, they have been found to allow increases in same-day exams, which can reduce the associated transportation-related emissions for patients compared to having to return on another date for imaging.

The 2014 RAND Corporation report on the Medicare Imaging Demonstration, deemed by the US FDA as one of the superior estimates for imaging appropriateness, found between 4% and 26% of CT and MR imaging studies evaluated overall were inappropriate, with inappropriateness of individual exam types estimated as high as 79% [30]. Calculated for only the US Medicare Part B population (28.6 million people total as of 2023), this inappropriate imaging generates up to 129.2 kT $CO_2$ equivalent per year (with up to 33.8 kT from MRI and 64.8 kT from CT) [30, 31].

To date, the usage of this type of CDS is primarily keyword based at the time of order entry, with considerable room remaining to develop more intelligent and proactive CDS systems to make evidence-based recommendations in favor of or against specific imaging studies based on information as it is entered into the patient note or perhaps even as an ambient scribe is recording the conversation. In addition to reducing inappropriate exams, CDS can assist in rapidly directing clinicians when imaging is needed and what type of imaging is needed to get to the most accurate diagnosis in the most efficient manner, potentially allowing for shortening of hospital stays. Implementing actionable CDS into the clinical workflow will allow for optimization of appropriate imaging.

Additionally, CDS systems could also be developed to take energy expenditure of different exams into account and thereby guide clinicians toward lower-energy imaging modalities when diagnostically equivalent. For example, AI can recommend ultrasound over CT for certain indications, reducing ionizing radiation exposure and energy consumption. This type of guidance, however, must be primarily driven by the clinical utility of these exams to ensure that it does not result in a net increase in overall imaging (and thereby overall emissions) from selecting inferior or even inappropriate imaging examinations solely due to their lower emissions.

Many times, the vast amount of information available in the electronic medical record can itself hide simple yet important information that an AI-powered CDS system could highlight, such as the fact that a patient may have already had an imaging study to answer the clinical question at hand with no significant clinical change in the patient since the time of that prior exam. Beyond this, an AI assistant could further reduce unnecessary imaging by synthesizing relevant information from prior diagnostic evaluations; for example, though a patient may not have had a prior abdomen MRI for evaluation of their adrenal glands, it is quite possible that they could have been seen and adequately evaluated on a prior chest CT.

Clinical decision support models could also be beneficial in further optimizing the use of IV contrast. By assessing the pretest probability that contrast would provide additional information, a model could help guide which examinations could be effectively performed without contrast. Pixel-based algorithms could also benefit in this area by assessing the pre-contrast images during their acquisition to determine if there are findings that could benefit from further characterization via contrast administration. AI assistants such as these would not only reduce waste from unnecessary contrast administration but would also be able to flag instances where unanticipated IV contrast would be beneficial in preventing a patient callback to get an additional study.

### 4.3.8 Enhanced Diagnostic Accuracy and Reduced Rescanning

Another method by which AI models could reduce the overall volume of imaging is to reduce the need for repeat imaging. Repeat imaging can contribute to increased energy expenditure in several manners: increased emissions from outpatient transportation, increased length of stay for inpatients or emergency department patients, redundancy in reacquisition of previously obtained images, and possible needs to employ additional resources via sedation.

One such manner of reducing repeated imaging is simply through improvement in image quality to reduce nondiagnostic image acquisition. Previously mentioned denoising and image acquisition acceleration techniques are one path to doing so, as a quicker examination will be less prone to disruption by patient motion. However, algorithms could be specifically tailored to assess for and mitigate the effects of patient motion, both via analysis of the raw imaging data and via direct patient monitoring.

Additionally, further development of virtual post-contrast imaging, as mentioned previously, could be beneficial to forgo the need for bringing patients back to get repeat imaging such as for instances in which an abnormality is identified on non-contrast imaging that could potentially be further characterized with IV contrast. Conceptually, this same type of algorithm development could be used to generate additional imaging using only the data that was already obtained. This could be useful not only in preventing rescanning in cases where additional MRI sequences could be beneficial but also in generating synthetic images of an entirely different modality based on the preexisting imaging data for that patient, such as generating a virtual CT scan from MRI images. Recent work in this area has shown the feasibility of deep learning models that generate synthetic CT from MRI for radiotherapy planning [32, 33], with further reviews highlighting broader applications of cross-modality image synthesis in radiology [34]. Commercial software has also begun to provide clinical tools for virtual CT generation from MRI data [35].

Alternatively, or perhaps alongside these methods for AI-based synthesis of images, AI models could be at the point of image acquisition to immediately determine and flag when additional imaging is needed, such as post-contrast imaging, additional MRI sequences, or even simply increases in anatomical coverage. Adding on such imaging at the time of the initial scan could provide significant savings in emissions, though this would need to be balanced appropriately and may require a human-in-the-loop approach to ensure that it would not end up lengthening scan times without clinical benefit.

## 4.4 Conclusion

Radiology's environmental footprint is a pressing concern, but AI presents viable pathways toward sustainability. While AI itself requires significant energy, its strategic application in workflow optimization, diagnostic precision, and imaging efficiency can lead to net reductions in resource consumption. Many such use cases also have potential for significant cost savings, both through direct decreases in energy expenditures and via downstream effects such as increasing revenue related to optimizing patient throughput or decreasing costs by using software to achieve results comparable to higher-end hardware. To fully realize AI's potential for reducing radiology's environmental footprint, sustainability must be integrated into every stage of adoption. Radiology has an opportunity not only to improve patient care but also to help lead medicine's broader shift toward a low-carbon future. Equally important is fostering awareness and education among radiologists—embedding sustainability principles into training, sharing evidence on measurable energy savings, and equipping clinicians with tools to track their own impact—so that AI-driven solutions are both implemented and actively championed by those on the front lines of imaging.

## References

1. Chaban YV, Vosshenrich J, McKee H, Gunasekaran S, Brown MJ, Atalay MK, et al. Environmental sustainability and MRI: challenges, opportunities, and a call for action. Magn Reson Imaging. 2024;59(4):1149–67.
2. Doo FX, Vosshenrich J, Cook TS, Moy L, Almeida EPRP, Woolen SA, et al. Environmental sustainability and AI in radiology: a double-edged sword. Radiology. 2024;310(2):e232030.
3. Health Care Without Harm, Arup. Health care's climate footprint: How the health sector contributes to the global climate crisis and opportunities

for action [Internet]. 2019 [cited 2025 Apr 24]. Available from: https://global.noharm.org/sites/default/files/documents-files/5961/HealthCaresClimateFootprint_092319.pdf

4. Schoen J, McGinty GB, Quirk C. Radiology in our changing climate: a call to action. J Am Coll Radiol. 2021;18(7):1041–3.
5. Brown M, Schoen JH, Gross J, Omary RA, Hanneman K. Climate change and radiology: impetus for change and a toolkit for action. Radiology. 2023;307(4):e230229.
6. Eckelman MJ, Sherman J. Environmental impacts of the U.S. health care system and effects on public health. Ahmad S, editor. PLoS One. 2016;11(6):e0157014.
7. Buckley BW, MacMahon PJ. Radiology and the climate crisis: opportunities and challenges—*radiology* in training. Radiology. 2021;300(3):E339–41.
8. Martin M, Mohnke A, Lewis GM, Dunnick NR, Keoleian G, Maturen KE. Environmental impacts of abdominal imaging: a pilot investigation. J Am Coll Radiol. 2018;15(10):1385–93.
9. Merkle EM, Bamberg F, Vosshenrich J. The impact of modern imaging techniques on carbon footprints: relevance and outlook. Eur Urol Focus. 2023;9(6):891–3.
10. Roletto A, Zanardo M, Bonfitto GR, Catania D, Sardanelli F, Zanoni S. The environmental impact of energy consumption and carbon emissions in radiology departments: a systematic review. Eur Radiol Exp. 2024;8(1):35.
11. Medical Imaging Equipment Version 1 | ENERGY STAR [Internet]. [cited 2025 Mar 31]. Available from: https://www.energystar.gov/products/spec/medical_imaging_equipment_version_1_0_pd
12. Prasanna PM, Siegel E, Kunce A. Greening radiology. J Am Coll Radiol. 2011;8(11):780–4.
13. Thaqi R, Kadriu M, Krasniqi B, Rexha B. On-premises versus cloud computing: a comparative analysis of energy consumption. In: 2024 International Conference on Renewable Energies and Smart Technologies (REST) [Internet]; 2024. p. 1–5. [cited 2025 Apr 2]. Available from: https://ieeexplore.ieee.org/abstract/document/10645419.
14. IEA [Internet]. [cited 2025 Apr 2]. Tracking clean energy progress 2023—analysis. Available from: https://www.iea.org/reports/tracking-clean-energy-progress-2023
15. Patterson D, Gonzalez J, Le Q, Liang C, Munguia LM, Rothchild D, et al. Carbon emissions and large neural network training [Internet]. arXiv. 2021; [cited 2025 Apr 1]. Available from: http://arxiv.org/abs/2104.10350
16. Center for Research on Foundation Models. OpenAI GPT-4 [Internet]. Stanford HAI; 2024 May [cited 2025 Apr 24]. Available from: https://crfm.stanford.edu/fmti/May-2024/company-reports/OpenAI_GPT-4.html

17. Energy Consumption of ChatGPT Responses | Baeldung on Computer Science [Internet]. 2024 [cited 2025 Apr 1]. Available from: https://www.baeldung.com/cs/chatgpt-large-language-models-power-consumption
18. Erdil E, Epoch AI. How has DeepSeek improved the Transformer architecture? [cited 2025 Mar 27]; 2025. Available from: https://epoch.ai/gradient-updates/how-has-deepseek-improved-the-transformer-architecture
19. Baidu Inc. Baidu Unveils ERNIE 4.5 and Reasoning Model ERNIE X1, Makes ERNIE Bot Free Ahead of Schedule [Internet]. [cited 2025 Mar 27]. Available from: https://www.prnewswire.com/news-releases/baidu-unveils-ernie-4-5-and-reasoning-model-ernie-x1%2D%2Dmakes-ernie-bot-free-ahead-of-schedule-302402490.html
20. Woolen SA, Becker AE, Martin AJ, et al. Ecodesign and operational strategies to reduce the carbon footprint of MRI for energy cost savings. Radiology. 2023;307(4):e230441.
21. McKee H, Brown MJ, Kim HHR, Doo FX, Panet H, Rockall AG, et al. Planetary health and radiology: why we should care and what we can do. Radiology. 2024;311(1):e240219.
22. Walters R, McAlister S, Dey C, Patlas MN. Reducing the carbon footprint of radiology through automatic workstation shutdown protocols. Eur Radiol. 2024;34(7):4710–8.
23. Rockall AG. The Green Radiology Department. EMJ Radiol. 2022;3(1):64–6. Available from: https://www.emjreviews.com/wp-content/uploads/2022/06/The-Green-Radiology-Department-1.pdf
24. Büttner L, Posch H, Auer TA, Jonczyk M, Fehrenbach U, Hamm B, et al. Switching off for future—Cost estimate and a simple approach to improving the ecological footprint of radiological departments. Eur J Radiol Open. 2020;8:100320.
25. Rockall AG, Allen B, Brown MJ, El-Diasty T, Fletcher J, Gerson RF, et al. Sustainability in radiology: position paper and call to action from ACR, AOSR, ASR, CAR, CIR, ESR, ESRNM, ISR, IS3R, RANZCR, and RSNA. Radiology. 2025;314(3):e250325.
26. Kagoma Y, Stall N, Rubinstein E, Naudie D. People, planet and profits: the case for greening operating rooms. CMAJ. 2012;184(17):1905–11.
27. Pasquini L, Napolitano A, Pignatelli M, Tagliente E, Parrillo C, Nasta F, et al. Synthetic post-contrast imaging through artificial intelligence: clinical applications of virtual and augmented contrast media. Pharmaceutics. 2022;14(11):2378.
28. NetZeroAICT Consortium. NetZeroAICT: Digital contrast for computerised tomography. Horizon Europe-funded research project (Grant No. 101136679); project webpage, 2025 [cited 2025 Aug 20]. Available from: https://netzeroaict.eu/
29. CareSelect® Imaging [Internet]. [cited 2025 Mar 31]. Available from: https://business.optum.com/en/operations-technology/clinical-decision-support/careselect/imaging.html

30. Cavanagh G, Schoen JH, Hanneman K, Rula EY, Atalay MK. Excess greenhouse gas emissions associated with inappropriate medical imaging in the US medicare Part B population from 2017 to 2021. J Am Coll Radiol [Internet]. 2025; [cited 2025 Mar 31];0(0). Available from: https://www.jacr.org/article/S1546-1440(25)00148-6/fulltext
31. Harvey L. Medicare beneficiary enrollment numbers: a research tool [Internet]. Neiman Health Policy Institute; 2020. [cited 2025 Mar 31]. Available from: https://www.neimanhpi.org/medicare-beneficiary-enrollment-tool/
32. MVision AI. Deep learning to generate synthetic CT images from MR for radiotherapy treatment planning [Internet]. 2023 [cited 2025 Aug 20]. Available from: https://mvision.ai/deep-learning-to-generate-synthetic-ct-images-from-mr-for-radiotherapy-treatment-planning/
33. Han X. MR-based synthetic CT generation using a deep convolutional neural network method. Med Phys. 2017;44(4):1408–19. Available from: https://pmc.ncbi.nlm.nih.gov/articles/PMC8166621/
34. Arif M, Kötter T, Kleesiek J, Isensee F, Maier-Hein KH, Kickingereder P, et al. Cross-modality image synthesis in radiology: a review. Insights Imaging. 2023;14:37. Available from: https://insightsimaging.springeropen.com/articles/10.1186/s13244-023-01603-6
35. MRIGuidance. BoneMRI—Virtual CT from MRI [Internet]. 2025 [cited 2025 Aug 20]. Available from: https://mriguidance.com/

# 5 Energy-Efficient AI Models and Sustainable Data Management Practices

Ángel Alberich-Bayarri, Ana Jiménez-Pastor, and Jose Munuera

## 5.1 Introduction

Artificial intelligence (AI) is transforming healthcare by enabling predictive diagnostics, automated workflows, and personalized treatments. However, the environmental cost of AI, especially in model training and large-scale data storage, is becoming a growing concern. The third wave of AI ethics emphasizes not only fairness and transparency but also environmental responsibility as a key component of sustainable development.

AI ethics has evolved through three major waves [1], each focusing on different challenges:

– First Wave: This wave was concerned with what AI might do in the future, especially the risks of superintelligence. Think of this phase as speculative and philosophical, exploring scenarios where AI could surpass human intelligence and pose existential risks.

Á. Alberich-Bayarri (✉) · A. Jiménez-Pastor · J. Munuera
Quibim, Valencia, Spain
e-mail: angel@quibim.com; anajimenez@quibim.com; josemunuera@quibim.com





E. R. Ranschaert et al. (eds.), *Sustainability of AI in Radiology*, Imaging Informatics for Healthcare Professionals,
https://doi.org/10.1007/978-3-032-15693-8_5

- Second Wave: As AI became more widely used, this wave addressed practical and immediate concerns related to machine learning. Key issues included the "black-box" nature of algorithms (making their decisions hard to explain), bias in training data that leads to unfair or discriminatory outcomes, and the increasing use of facial and emotion recognition technologies that could infringe on individual rights.
- Third Wave: The most recent wave shifts focus to the environmental impact of AI. It tackles the significant energy consumption and carbon footprint of training large models. This wave aims to bring together researchers, policymakers, developers, and the public to build awareness and solutions for AI's role in the climate crisis. Healthcare presents a unique case: while AI promises to reduce diagnostic error, personalize treatment, and improve efficiency, the carbon emissions resulting from model training and continuous inference workflows can offset its benefits if not managed responsibly.

In medical imaging, AI plays a central role in tasks such as segmentation, classification, detection, and prognosis, bringing improvements in speed, accuracy, and scalability. Deep learning architectures, especially convolutional neural networks (CNNs), U-Net variants for image segmentation, vision transformers (ViTs), and hybrid 3D models, have become foundational in this domain. These architectures have been instrumental in advancing applications ranging from tumor detection in radiology to organ segmentation and radiomics-based biomarker discovery.

Major technology and health companies such as Google Health, IBM Watson Health, Siemens Healthineers, GE Healthcare, and Philips have invested heavily in developing AI-driven solutions for medical imaging. At the same time, rising AI-native players like Aidoc, Viz.ai, Quibim, HeartFlow, and Corti are pushing innovation through purpose-built AI platforms. These companies integrate AI not only into diagnosis and triage but also into workflow optimization and population health management.

However, as the adoption of AI in healthcare accelerates, so does its environmental footprint. Training state-of-the-art models, particularly large-scale vision and transformer-based networks, or the so-called foundation models, where deep networks with billions of parameters and millions of data samples are trained, can emit substantial amounts of $CO_2$. According to Strubell et al. [2], training a single large natural language processing model can produce as much carbon as five cars over their entire lifetimes, a figure that, although domain-specific, points to a critical issue across AI disciplines.

The third wave of AI ethics extends the discussion beyond bias, fairness, and transparency to include environmental sustainability as a core ethical concern. This shift is particularly relevant in healthcare, where the tension between innovation and responsibility is pronounced. Surprisingly, while ethical AI is a growing topic, few companies in healthcare AI explicitly report on the sustainability of their models or infrastructure. Some academic initiatives and policy think tanks, such as the Alan Turing Institute, Stanford's Center for Biomedical Ethics, and MIT's Schwarzman College of Computing, are beginning to incorporate environmental dimensions into the ethical evaluation of AI. Still, sustainability reporting in this field remains sparse and largely voluntary.

This chapter explores the tools, strategies, and ethical frameworks that support energy-efficient AI model development and sustainable data practices. We discuss model compression techniques (such as pruning, quantization, and knowledge distillation), sustainable hardware choices, green data center partnerships, and responsible data life cycle management. Through a combination of technical strategies and case studies, we highlight how institutions and companies can adopt greener practices without compromising innovation.

## 5.2 Environmental Impact of AI Development

Training state-of-the-art AI models, such as large language models or deep neural networks for medical imaging, is computationally intensive. For instance, training GPT-3 consumed an estimated

1287 MWh, equivalent to the annual electricity consumption of over 120 US households [3]. In healthcare, imaging-based AI models often require massive annotated datasets and long training cycles, further amplifying energy use.

Training large-scale AI models can produce massive carbon emissions. Strubell et al. [2] estimated that training a large NLP model could result in over 272,16 metric tonnes of $CO_2$ emissions. Google's AlphaGo Zero reportedly generated 96 tonnes of $CO_2$ in just 40 days of training [1]. Such statistics underscore the need for sustainable practices in model training.

The underlying causes include the need for high-performance computing resources, extended training times, and nonrenewable energy sources. With over 600 million people globally lacking access to modern electricity, there is a clear ethical tension between AI development and global energy equity. A summary of relevant AI architectures and associated energy consumption and carbon emissions is provided in Table 5.1.

The global distribution of AI development is uneven. Most training occurs in regions with access to affordable computing and nonrenewable energy. In contrast, emerging economies often lack the infrastructure to compete. This creates ethical tensions, particularly when AI applications are deployed in low-resource settings without corresponding local development or energy offsets.

In addition to carbon emissions, AI model training and inference also incur hidden environmental costs, particularly in water consumption. Data centers, which power both model training and large-scale image generation, require significant amounts of water for cooling. According to recent estimates, generating just 20 images using AI models like the popular Ghibli-style trend on platforms such as MidJourney or Stable Diffusion can consume a non-negligible amount of liters of clean water when accounting for both direct and indirect cooling processes [4].

At scale, the numbers are staggering. A single AI training run for a large model can consume millions of liters of water, often sourced from municipal supplies during peak demand hours. For example, research from the University of California, Riverside, suggests that training GPT-3 may have used 700,000 liters

**Table 5.1** MIT technology review

| | Date of original paper | Energy consumption (kWh) | Carbon footprint (tonnes of $CO_2e$) | Cloud compute cost (USD) |
|---|---|---|---|---|
| Transformer (65 M parameters) | Jun, 2017 | 27 | 0.01 | \$41–\$140 |
| Transformer (213 M parameters) | Jun, 2017 | 201 | 0.09 | \$289–\$981 |
| ELMo | Feb, 2018 | 275 | 0.12 | \$433–\$1472 |
| BERT (110 M parameters) | Oct, 2018 | 1507 | 0.65 | \$3751–\$12,571 |
| Transformer (213 M parameters) with neural architecture search | Jan, 2019 | 656,347 | 284.02 | \$942,973–\$3,201,722 |
| GPT-2 | Feb, 2019 | – | – | \$12,902–\$43,008 |

Source: [2]
Note: Because of a lack of power draw data on GPT-2's training hardware, the researchers weren't able to calculate its carbon footprint

(184,000 gallons) of freshwater, primarily for cooling the servers (Li et al., 2023). These water demands are typically concentrated in areas already facing climate stress or drought risk, further intensifying ethical concerns around AI's resource footprint.

While some hyperscale data centers employ closed-loop cooling systems that recirculate water, these systems are not entirely self-sufficient. In practice, water is lost through evaporation in cooling towers and must be replenished regularly. In temperate climates, air-based or hybrid cooling can reduce water usage, but in hotter regions, evaporative cooling is often more efficient and thus more water-intensive.

Moreover, although many providers claim Artificial intelligence (AI) to reuse or recycle water [5], the quality of reused water often degrades over cycles, and additional treatment is required, limiting how many times water can be effectively recirculated. As a result, even "efficient" data centers still consume significant volumes of freshwater, particularly during high-demand periods like training large AI models or supporting viral image-generation trends.

## 5.3 Tools and Metrics for Sustainability

Evaluating the sustainability of AI systems requires robust tools and metrics to track and mitigate their environmental impact. The number of tools and methodologies available for assessing the carbon footprint, energy consumption, and broader environmental costs of AI systems is growing, and some of them are increasingly being used by companies that need to fulfill their environmental, social, and governance (ESG) goals [6], including low $CO_2$ emissions:

1. Machine Learning Emissions Calculator: This tool estimates the carbon footprint of AI models by considering compute time, hardware specifications, and the geographic location of data centers, which affects the energy grid's carbon intensity [7].
2. Carbontracker: Carbontracker provides real-time tracking of energy consumption during training cycles, enabling researchers to estimate emissions and identify opportunities for optimization [8].
3. Experiment-impact-tracker: This tool offers visual reporting of emissions data and helps researchers generate standardized appendices for academic papers, ensuring transparency in reporting sustainability metrics [9].
4. HaraAI: HaraAI is a method that proposes token-based metrics to estimate computational complexity and track emissions from AI models. This approach leverages existing data on token usage in APIs to provide a granular understanding of carbon emissions [10].
5. SKD4ED: This tool evaluates energy efficiency during software development processes, enabling organizations to optimize their workflows for reduced energy consumption [11].

6. CodeCarbon: CodeCarbon is an open-source software package that seamlessly integrates into Python-based algorithms. It estimates the emissions and energy consumption produced by the cloud or personal computing resources used to execute the code [12].

Some of the metrics usually reported for sustainability assessment are the following:

- Carbon-related metrics such as $CO_2$ equivalent ($CO_2e$) emissions are used to measure the environmental impact of AI systems throughout their life cycle, including training, deployment, and hardware manufacturing. Common metrics:
  - $CO_2e$ emissions (kg or tons): Total carbon dioxide equivalent emissions
  - Emissions per training run (e.g., GPT-3 ~ 96 $tCO_2e$)
  - $CO_2e$ per inference/query
  - Carbon intensity of energy used ($gCO_2$/kWh)
- Energy Consumption: Evaluates how much electricity is required to train, fine-tune, and run AI models. Common metrics:
  - Total energy used (kWh or MWh) for training
  - Energy per training epoch
  - Energy per inference (joules/query).
  - Power usage effectiveness (PUE) of data centers
- Water Usage: Metrics that account for water consumption in cooling data centers are increasingly being integrated into sustainability assessments. Common metrics:
  - Liters or gallons of water used per training run
  - Water usage effectiveness (WUE) = liters/kWh
  - Direct vs. indirect water usage (e.g., from electricity generation)
  - Evaporative losses in cooling towers
- Life Cycle Analysis: Comprehensive life cycle assessments consider not only the operational phase but also the manufacturing and end-of-life phases of hardware used in AI systems. Common metrics:
  - Embodied carbon in hardware (kg $CO_2e$)
  - Device lifespan vs. utilization rate

- E-waste generated
- Environmental impact per model life cycle phase

## 5.4 Strategies for Energy-Efficient AI

AI systems have become increasingly resource-intensive, necessitating strategies to improve energy efficiency. These strategies span algorithmic optimizations, hardware advancements, and deployment practices. The energy-efficient AI approaches can be classified as algorithmic, hardware-based, and deployment related:

### 5.4.1 Algorithmic Strategies

Trained deep networks require extensive computer power not only during training but also on inference, imposing large energy demands. Table 5.2 shows the hardware requirements to run some of the open-source LLMs used for daily tasks. These models are frequently adapted to create healthcare-specialized variants, such as MedAlpaca and ClinicalCamel, which are derived from different versions of the LLaMA models.

Different strategies can be followed to reduce the complexity and size of these trained models to improve their efficiency in both execution time and energy requirements. Some of the most common strategies are the following (Fig. 5.1):

- Pruning

Pruning simplifies AI models by removing unnecessary components, such as redundant weights or neurons, thereby reducing computational overhead.

- Magnitude-Based Pruning: Removes weights with the smallest magnitudes, assuming they contribute minimally to model performance. This technique reduces model complexity while preserving accuracy [13].

**Table 5.2** List of some of the commonly known LLMs used for different daily tasks

| Model | Parameters (billion, B) | Estimated hardware requirements (inference) | Publication year |
|---|---|---|---|
| DeepSeek-VL | 7B / 67B | 7B: 1x RTX 3090/4090<br>67B: 4-8x A100 80GB | 2024 |
| DeepSeek-Coder | 6.7B / 33B | 6.7B: 1x RTX 3090/4090<br>33B: 2-4x A100 80GB | 2024 |
| Qwen | 7B / 14B | 7B: 1x GPU 16GB<br>14B: 1-2x GPU 24-40GB | 2023 |
| Mistral | 7B | 1x GPU 12-16GB | 2023 |
| LLaMA 2 | 7B / 13B / 70B | 7B: 1x GPU 16GB<br>13B: 1x GPU 24 GB<br>70B: 4x A100 80GB | 2023 |
| Phi-2 | 2.7B | CPU or small GPU | 2023 |

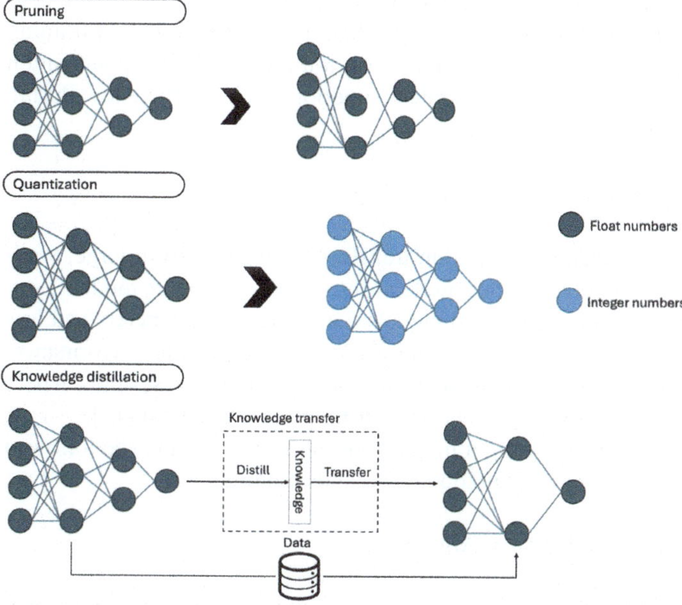


**Fig. 5.1** Strategies to reduce the complexity and size of trained AI models

- Structured Pruning: Eliminates entire structural components like filters or layers, leading to significant reductions in computational costs and memory usage. Structured pruning is particularly effective for convolutional neural networks (CNNs) deployed on resource-constrained devices.
- Iterative Pruning: Gradually removes support vectors or neurons while retraining the model to minimize accuracy loss. This iterative approach ensures optimal balance between efficiency and performance.

- Quantization

Quantization reduces the precision of numerical values in computations, such as transitioning from 32-bit floating-point numbers to 8-bit integers. This technique significantly lowers memory and compute demand without substantial accuracy degradation. Emerging methods like gradient-based post-training quantization (GPTQ) and activation-aware weight quantization (AWQ) have demonstrated superior energy efficiency during inference phases [14].

- Knowledge Distillation

Knowledge distillation transfers knowledge from large, complex models (teacher models) into smaller, simpler models (student models). Distilled models require fewer parameters and less computational power while achieving comparable performance. Applications include real-time decision-making systems where reduced latency and energy consumption are critical [15].

However, during training, some strategies can also be followed to minimize computational demands required:

- Energy-Efficient Algorithms

Algorithmic changes that reduce the number of computational steps or operations can contribute significantly to energy savings. For example, regularization techniques like dropout and weight decay during training improve generalization while reducing resource requirements during inference [16]. Also, strategies such as early stopping can end the process when the model's performance on a validation set stops improving, reducing the number of needed epochs and, in consequence, the time and energy consumed.

### 5.4.2 Hardware-Based Strategies

- Specialized Hardware Design
    - Application-Specific Integrated Circuits (ASICs): Custom-designed for specific AI workloads, ASICs minimize unnecessary overhead and maximize efficiency. Examples include Eyeriss chips tailored for deep learning tasks [17].
    - Field-Programmable Gate Arrays (FPGAs): Reconfigurable platforms optimized for specific AI tasks offer better energy efficiency compared to general-purpose processors [18].
- Low-Power Components
    - Low-power processors designed for mobile or IoT devices can reduce energy usage during training and inference phases [19].
    - Efficient memory hierarchies that minimize data movement and maximize data reuse further enhance hardware efficiency [20].
- Dynamic Voltage and Frequency Scaling (DVFS): Adapting the operating voltage and clock frequency of hardware components based on workload requirements can save energy when full utilization is unnecessary [21].
- Cooling and Thermal Management: Proper cooling solutions prevent overheating, which can lead to inefficiencies and reduced hardware lifespan. In temperate climates, air-based cooling systems can be employed to reduce water usage while maintaining operational efficiency [22].

### 5.4.3 Deployment Practices

- Carbon-Aware Cloud Platforms: Cloud providers are increasingly integrating carbon-aware options into their services, enabling users to optimize deployments based on renewable energy availability or lower-carbon grids such as Google's Carbon-Intelligent Computing Platform, which moves computing tasks between data centers based on regional hourly carbon-free energy availability [23, 24].
- Energy Monitoring Tools: Real-time monitoring systems like Carbontracker provide insights into energy consumption during training cycles, allowing researchers to dynamically optimize workloads based on energy constraints [8].
- Efficient Workload Management: Load balancing across multiple hardware components prevents overloading some components while underutilizing others, ensuring optimal resource usage at lower energy costs [25].

## 5.5 Sustainable Data Management

Data storage is a critical yet often-overlooked contributor to the environmental impact of AI. The vast amounts of data required for training, deploying, and operating AI models have led to exponential growth in storage demands. This growth is not without consequences, as data centers consume substantial energy and resources, contributing to greenhouse gas (GHG) emissions and environmental degradation.

One significant challenge is the accumulation of "dark data," which refers to data that is collected but never used. Estimates suggest that over half of an organization's stored data falls into this category, consuming energy without delivering any operational or analytical value [26]. This inefficiency exacerbates the environmental footprint of AI, especially as global data center power demand is projected to surge by 160% by 2030.

To mitigate these impacts, organizations can adopt several best practices:

- Cold Storage for Infrequently Accessed Archives: Cold storage solutions are designed for data that is rarely accessed, using energy-efficient systems that minimize power consumption. These systems are ideal for archiving historical datasets or backups that do not require immediate retrieval.
- Data Life cycle Management: Implementing robust data life cycle management policies ensures that obsolete or redundant datasets are identified and deleted. This approach not only reduces storage costs but also minimizes the energy required to maintain unused data.
- Duplicate Data Sample Detection: Another common issue in organizations' data storage is the presence of duplicated data, which not only impacts the carbon footprint but also can introduce biases if used for model training and not properly identified. A common method for duplicate detection involves applying hashing (e.g., SHA-256 or MD5) to records or files to identify exact duplicates. For near-duplicates, fuzzy matching techniques such as Levenshtein distance or Jaccard similarity can be used.
- Clean Energy-Powered Data Centers: Transitioning to renewable energy sources for powering data centers significantly reduces their carbon footprint. Companies like Google and Microsoft have already made strides in this area by integrating renewable energy into their operations. Google Cloud, for example, has matched all its annual electricity use with an equivalent amount of renewable energy since 2017, effectively powering its operations with clean energy on an annual basis.

AI itself can play a role in improving the sustainability of data storage. Advanced machine learning algorithms can optimize storage configurations dynamically based on workload demands, ensuring maximum efficiency while minimizing resource use. Additionally, AI tools can facilitate predictive maintenance for storage hardware, extending its lifespan and reducing electronic waste [27].

## 5.6 Case Studies from the Experience in Medical Imaging

Medical imaging represents a particularly relevant domain for developing energy-efficient AI systems. These applications often involve processing large, high-resolution scans, sometimes across multiple modalities or timepoints. Building models for classification, detection, or segmentation tasks typically demands significant computational resources and careful data pipeline management. While the clinical benefits of AI are increasingly well established, the environmental footprint associated with training and deploying such models should not be overlooked. In particular, the training phase is the most energy-demanding stage due to repeated passes over large datasets, the optimization of parameters, the use of complex architectures, and the multiple experiments that usually are performed until the best model is developed. With thoughtful design choices, however, this impact can be substantially reduced without compromising diagnostic accuracy. In addition to optimizing training, improving the energy efficiency of inference is also crucial, particularly for large-scale or real-time clinical deployments, where savings in energy needed per prediction can contribute to a significant environmental benefit.

This case study outlines several key strategies employed in the development of a classification model intended to identify active axial spondyloarthritis (axSpA) using MRI scans. Energy consumption metrics were measured with CodeCarbon.

Architectural Considerations: 2D vs. 3D Models

One of the initial design decisions involved selecting between a 2D and 3D model architecture. Each approach offers distinct advantages and trade-offs:

- **3D models** are capable of directly processing volumetric data, which allows them to capture rich spatial context across slices. However, they are computationally intensive, require more memory, and typically demand longer training times.

- **2D models**, by contrast, operate on individual image slices. Although this reduces their ability to model inter-slice relationships, it significantly lowers the computational cost of training and inference.

From an energy efficiency perspective, 2D models generally consume far fewer resources. In many cases, particularly when full volumetric context is not essential, they can offer comparable performance while dramatically reducing both training time and energy consumption.

### 5.6.1 Using Pretrained Encoders

Another important consideration was whether to train the model from scratch or initialize it with pretrained weights. The latter approach, which involves using encoders trained on large image datasets such as ImageNet [28] or domain-specific repositories like MedicalNet [29], offers substantial advantages in terms of both efficiency and performance.

By initializing the model with pretrained weights, early layers begin with a representation of generic visual features. This reduces the number of epochs required for convergence, resulting in a shorter training cycle and lower overall energy usage. The reuse of these pretrained components also encourages reproducibility and simplifies the development process, particularly valuable when computational resources are limited.

Early Stopping as a Regularization and Efficiency Tool

To avoid unnecessary computation and reduce the risk of overfitting, early stopping was implemented. This technique monitors validation performance during training and halts the process once improvements plateau. In practice, this often results in a substantial reduction in the number of training epochs, which in turn decreases GPU hours and energy use.

Although early stopping is a standard regularization method, its value from an energy efficiency standpoint is not always highlighted. In energy-conscious AI development, it represents a simple yet impactful strategy.

### 5.6.2 Model Training Experiments

Applying the strategies described above, a series of experiments was conducted to develop the classification model for axSpA. Both 2D and 3D approaches were explored, with all models initialized using pretrained weights and trained with early stopping criteria in place. Table 5.3 presents the results of the experiments that demonstrated the best performance across the evaluation metrics.

The experiments suggest that, for this particular case, the 2D models offered a more efficient solution in terms of energy consumption while still achieving strong performance. Using pretrained weights helped the models reach convergence in fewer training epochs than expected, and when paired with early stopping, this significantly shortened the training time. As a result, the overall energy used during model development was notably reduced without a loss in performance. This efficiency is relevant not only from a sustainability point of view but also from a financial one. The lower energy consumption needed by the models directly affects the cost of both training and deploying the final solution.

On the other hand, the 3D models generally took longer to train and required more computational power to reach similar results. This added to the energy cost and made them less practical for the given task. One example, referred to here as Model 3, failed to deliver acceptable performance and did not reach early stopping at all. While it did not meet expectations, it highlighted a common part of the development process: testing multiple configurations before arriving close to the expected results. These less successful runs can be particularly demanding in terms of energy, reinforcing the importance of making thoughtful design choices early on. In healthcare, where costs and accessibility are critical, this underlines the importance of selecting strategies that are not only accurate but also sustainable and affordable. The overarching goal should be to maximize clinical value while minimizing energy and financial cost, making AI more democratic and widely available.

**Table 5.3** Model development experiments for axSPa classification

| Model ID | Architecture | AUC (test) | Emissions (kWh) | Energy consumed (kWh) | GPU Energy (W) | Num Epochs | Training time |
|---|---|---|---|---|---|---|---|
| Model 1 | ResNet 2D | 0.94 | 0.33 | 1.52 | 1.15 | 52 (e.s.) | 3 h 17 min |
| Model 2 | ResNet 2D | 0.94 | 0.31 | 1.44 | 1.05 | 55 (e.s.) | 3 h 24 min |
| Model 3 | DualResNet 3D | 0.77 | 1.58 | 7.31 | 5.35 | 400 | 17 h 14 min |
| Model 4 | DualResNet 3D | 0.94 | 1.69 | 3.17 | 2.54 | 216 (e.s.) | 5 h 34 min |

## 5.7 Conclusion

The AI research community must move beyond performance benchmarks to also report environmental metrics. This includes emissions per epoch, training time, and inference efficiency. Institutions should mandate energy transparency in publications and invest in green infrastructure.

As AI continues to shape modern society, its environmental implications can no longer be overlooked. Energy-efficient models and sustainable data practices are essential for ethical, long-term deployment of AI. By prioritizing carbon awareness, the AI ecosystem can drive innovation while maintaining environmental stewardship.

**Conflicts of Interest** AAB is CEO and shareholder of Quibim.

**Disclosure** No generative AI tools have been used for the conceptualization or creation of this publication and associated materials, such as figures.

## References

1. van Wynsberghe A. Sustainable AI: AI for sustainability and the sustainability of AI. AI Ethics. 2021;1:213–8.
2. Strubell E, Ganesh A, McCallum A. Energy and policy considerations for deep learning in NLP. arXiv:1906.02243. 2019;
3. Li P, Yang J, Islam MA, Ren S. Making AI less "thirsty": uncovering and addressing the secret water footprint of AI models. arXiv: 2304.03271. 2025;
4. Bertazzini G, Albisani C, Baracchi D, Shullani D, Verdecchia R. The hidden cost of an image: quantifying the energy consumption of AI image generation. arXiv preprint arXiv:2506.17016. 2025;
5. World Economic Forum (2024) Circular water solutions for sustainable data centres. https://www.weforum.org/stories/2024/11/circular-water-solutions-sustainable-data-centres/. Accessed 1 Apr 2025.
6. Picard N, Kosar J. AI and transparency: a new age of corporate responsibility. https://www.pwc.com/gx/en/services/audit-assurance/corporate-reporting/esg-reporting/ai-transparency-and-corporate-responsibility.html. Accessed on 19 Aug 2025.
7. Lacoste A, Luccioni A, Schmidt V, Dandres T. Quantifying the carbon emissions of machine learning. arXiv:1910.09700. 2019;

8. Anthony LFW, Kanding B, Selvan R. Carbontracker: tracking and predicting the carbon footprint of training deep learning models. arXiv:2007.03051. 2020;
9. Masciari E, Napolitano, EV (2024). An effective measure for evaluating the environmental impact of Ai tasks. Available at SSRN: https://ssrn.com/abstract=4962273
10. People+AI (2024) HaraAI: understanding and tracking AI's environmental impact. https://peopleplus.ai/blog/haraai-understanding-and-tracking-ai-s-environmental-impact. Accessed 28 Mar 2025.
11. Marantos C, Salapas K, Papadopoulos L, Soudris D. A flexible tool for estimating applications performance and energy consumption through static analysis. SN Comput Sci. 2021;2:2021.
12. Courty B, Schmidt V, Kamal G, Coutarel M, et al. mlco2/codecarbon: v2.4.1. Zenodo. 2024;
13. Kamolov S. Optimizing model pruning for energy-efficient deep learning. Ann Math Comput Sci. 2024;25:112–9.
14. Rajput S, Sharma T. Benchmarking emerging deep learning quantization methods for energy efficiency. In: IEEE 21st international conference on software architecture companion (ICSA-C), Hyderabad, India, 2024; 2024. p. 238–42. https://doi.org/10.1109/ICSA-C63560.2024.00049.
15. Yuan Y, Shi J, Zhang Z, Chen K, Zhang J, Stoico V, Malavolta I. The impact of knowledge distillation on the energy consumption and runtime efficiency of NLP models. In: Proceedings of the IEEE/ACM 3rd international conference on AI engineering - software engineering for AI (CAIN '24). Association for Computing Machinery, New York, NY, USA; 2024. p. 129–33. https://doi.org/10.1145/3644815.3644966.
16. Penev K, Gegov A, Isiaq O, Jafari R. Energy efficiency evaluation of artificial intelligence algorithms. Electronics. 2024;13(19):3836. https://doi.org/10.3390/electronics13193836.
17. Ahsan SMM, Dhungel A, Chowdhury M, Hasan MS, Hoque T. Hardware Accelerators for Artificial Intelligence. arXiv preprint arXiv. 2024:2411.13717.
18. Boutros A, Arora A, Betz V. Field-programmable gate Array architecture for deep learning: survey & future directions. arXiv preprint arXiv:2404.10076. 2024;
19. Georgios S. Low-power AI chips: empowering the next generation of intelligent devices. Int J Adv Innovat Thoughts Ideas. 2024;12:308. https://doi.org/10.4172/2277-1891.1000307.
20. Desislavov R, Martínez-Plumed F, Hernández-Orallo J. Trends in AI inference energy consumption: beyond the performance-vs-parameter laws of deep learning. Sustain Comput Inform Syst. 2023;38:100857. ISSN 2210–5379
21. Cardoso J, Coutinho JGF, Diniz PC. Chapter 2: High-performance embedded computing. In: Cardoso J, JGF C, Diniz PC, editors. Embedded computing for high performance. Morgan Kaufmann; 2017. p. 17–56.

ISBN 9780128041895. https://doi.org/10.1016/B978-0-12-804189-5.00002-8.

22. Chang Q, Huang Y, Liu K, Xu X, Zhao Y, Pan S. Optimization control strategies and evaluation metrics of cooling systems in data centers: a review. Sustainability. 2024;16(16):7222. https://doi.org/10.3390/su16167222.
23. Buchanan W, Foxon J, Cooke D, Iyer S, Graham E, DeRusha B, Binder C, Chiu K, Corso L, Richardson H, Knight V, Hussain A, Allison A, Mathews N. Carbon-aware computing. Measuring and reducing the carbon intensity associated with software in execution. Green Software Foundation (GSF); 2023.
24. Patel P, Gregersen T, Anderson T. An agile pathway towards carbon-aware clouds. SIGENERGY Energy Inform Rev. 2024;4(3):10–7. https://doi.org/10.1145/3698365.3698368.
25. Lilhore UK, Simaiya S, Prajapati YN, Rai AK, Ghith ES, Tlija M, Lamoudan T, Abdelhamid AA. A multi-objective approach to load balancing in cloud environments integrating ACO and WWO techniques. Sci Rep. 2025;15:12036. https://doi.org/10.1038/s41598-025-96364-1.
26. Jackson T, Hodgkinson I. Why, where and when dark data affects greenhouse gas emissions. Loughborough University; 2024. https://acss.org.uk/wp-content/uploads/IAG-briefing-dark-data-and-greenhouse-gas-emissions.pdf. Accessed 29 Mar 2025
27. Henry J, Halil M. Sustainable data storage for AI applications: securing critical information for environmental responsibility. EasyChair Preprint.12214; 2024. https://easychair.org/publications/preprint/26wXb. Accessed 30 Mar 2025
28. Deng J, Dong W, Socher R, Li LJ, Li K, Fei-Fei L. Imagenet: a large-scale hierarchical image database. In: 2009 IEEE conference on computer vision and pattern recognition. IEEE; 2009, June. p. 248–55.
29. Chen S, Ma K, Zheng Y. Med3d: transfer learning for 3d medical image analysis. arXiv preprint arXiv:1904.00625. 2019;

# 6 Patients and the Public: Sustainability and AI in Radiology

John Kellas and David Taylor

## 6.1 Introduction

This chapter explores three interrelated themes in radiological innovation: trust in AI, public engagement, and environmental sustainability. It examines the pivotal role of patient and public involvement (PPIE) in fostering transparency and accountability, ensuring that advances in radiology not only enhance diagnostic and clinical outcomes but also align with societal values and ecological imperatives.

John Kellas, lead author of this chapter, and contributing author David Taylor—who authored "AIM (*AI in Medicine*) and the Patient's Perspective" [1], are advocates for integrating patient and public perspectives into the research and development of health AI. Kellas, an expert in health informatics literacy and public involvement in AI, bridges the gap between complex healthcare technologies and the communities they serve. He is currently

J. Kellas (✉)
Nuffield Department of Surgical Sciences, University of Oxford, Oxford, UK
e-mail: john.kellas@nds.ox.ac.uk

D. Taylor
Digital Health Council, Royal Society of Medicine, London, UK



E. R. Ranschaert et al. (eds.), *Sustainability of AI in Radiology*, Imaging Informatics for Healthcare Professionals,
https://doi.org/10.1007/978-3-032-15693-8_6

a DPhil researcher at the University of Oxford, leading stakeholder engagement for the NetZero AICT project and facilitating public involvement for national and regional UK data research initiatives. Taylor, recently retired from Imperial College London, now serves as a patient representative in various healthcare research projects and underscores the critical importance of public trust in healthcare innovation, stating that "public trust in the industry is essential to realise the AI-enabled health data economy" [1]. The use of generative AI (Perplexity, ChatGPT, and Google Gemini) was used for assistance in research, drafting, and editing of this chapter.

Involving and engaging patients and the public in health AI research is fundamental to ensuring quality assurance, regulatory compliance, and widespread acceptance. Good PPIE fosters active partnerships between patients, the public, and professionals in health and social care research, driving meaningful improvements [2]. As stated in a 2022 joint statement by the UK's Medicines and Healthcare products Regulatory Agency (MHRA), National Institute for Health and Care Research (NIHR), and Health Research Authority (HRA): "Public involvement is important, expected, and possible in all types of health and social care research" [3]. Public involvement goes beyond one-way communication strategies to include co-investigation, co-design, co-production, and co-management. Unfortunately, public and patient involvement in health AI research is rare, or at least it is rarely reported. A 2024 scoping review found that, of 10,880 articles describing AI healthcare applications, only 21 (0.2%) described community involvement outside of an academic hospital setting [4].

The European Environment Agency emphasises that public participation is not only a matter of justice and democracy but also a practical necessity for transitioning to sustainability [5]. An inclusive approach ensures that advancements are grounded in real-world concerns, fostering trust and innovation. As Hannah Russell of the British Science Association's Sciencewise programme asserts, "When you bring together the public with researchers—that's when the magic happens. Bringing people into the conversation makes for better science" [6].

Citizen advocacy has played a pivotal role in raising the profile of climate concerns and driving policy change. Public attitude trackers show broad support for stronger climate action, indicating a deep and widespread concern that transcends national and economic boundaries. Social activist movements like Extinction Rebellion (XR) further demonstrate the strength of sentiment and public valuation of sustainability. As AI continues to evolve, understanding and incorporating patient perspectives is not only an ethical responsibility but also strategically important for building trust and achieving equitable, sustainable healthcare outcomes.

## 6.2 The Critical Role of Trust and Acceptance in AI

Public confidence in AI-driven radiology is built on a foundation of trust. While AI holds great promise for enhancing radiological practices, concerns about ethics, safety, equity, and transparency persist [7]. But how can AI projects earn public trust? What contributes to public trust and acceptance of AI technologies?

The European Commission's High-Level Expert Group on AI proposed Ethics Guidelines for Trustworthy AI [8], with foundational elements—lawfulness, ethics, and robustness—structured around key requirements: human agency and oversight; technical robustness and safety; privacy and data governance; transparency; diversity, non-discrimination, and fairness; societal and environmental well-being; and accountability [8]. AI research and development projects and products must adhere to the General Data Protection Regulation (GDPR) and other regulatory frameworks. Still, these frameworks do not necessarily reflect the tacit requirements for social acceptance. Public trust in research, innovation pipelines, and AI-driven radiology applications cannot be assumed [9] nor can we take for granted that expectations will be met [10].

Hannah Russell highlights that what the public cares about most includes "who governs the technology, who benefits from the technology, and whether the technology is safe and secure"

[6]. Addressing these concerns transparently fosters public trust in AI-driven healthcare advancements.

Where AI research projects have not had any patient or public involvement, friction and inertia in research translation are more likely further down the line. As the proverb goes, "If you want to go fast, go alone; if you want to go far, go together."

The UK Government's Public Attitudes to Data & AI Tracker (Wave 4) and The Health Foundation [11] show mixed comfort levels and highlight that familiarity, explainability, governance, and fairness strongly influence trust [11, 12].

In a recent systematic review of stakeholder perspectives on clinical AI implementation [9], the authors highlight an under-representation of non-Health Care Professional stakeholder perspectives, which may limit anticipation and management of implementation factors.

Transparency and accountability are also vital to building trust. As Taylor notes, "Open dialogue with the public is essential" [1]. This dialogue must address concerns such as the security of personal health data, ethical use of AI, equitable access to benefits, and protection from risks. Explainability, acceptability, accountability, and equity are all important dimensions of trust. Regulatory requirements do not always reflect the true social licence required for public acceptance.

## 6.3 Public Awareness and Understanding of AI

Despite its growing prevalence in healthcare, public understanding of AI remains limited. Taylor highlights that "citizens are often unaware of the importance of data sharing for AI research and development" [1]. Misunderstandings about AI's capabilities, sometimes fuelled by sensationalist media coverage, can exacerbate scepticism and fear. Recent national surveys indicate a significant gap between awareness of AI in general and understanding of its specific applications in healthcare [11, 12].

Simplifying complex technical concepts and showcasing real-world success stories can help bridge this understanding gap. For example, co-designed public workshops and informational campaigns can explain how AI supports diagnostic accuracy and safety in radiology. Taylor argues that preparing the public for widespread AI adoption requires concerted efforts from government, healthcare providers, and technologists. Transparent communication and accessible educational resources can empower patients to make informed decisions and foster greater acceptance of AI in healthcare.

Public awareness efforts can both address knowledge gaps about AI's potential benefits and proactively attend to governance, safety, and equitable impacts—including environmental and economic—to bridge the gap between researchers and the communities they serve.

## 6.4 Addressing Concerns and Fears

Public concerns about AI frequently revolve around data privacy, ethical risks, and algorithmic reliability. High-profile controversies, such as the Royal Free London–DeepMind data sharing arrangements, have heightened fears about transparency and potential misuse of sensitive health data [13, 14, 24]. As Taylor notes, "Opaque practices erode trust and lead to backlash, underscoring the need for candour in data sharing" [1].

Data privacy remains a significant barrier to AI acceptance. Patients worry about who has access to their medical information and how it might be used. Ensuring that AI systems adhere to strict data protection standards and involve clear, informed consent processes is critical.

Ethical risks—such as bias in training datasets—and algorithmic reliability further compound public fears. These biases can lead to inequities in healthcare outcomes, disproportionately affecting marginalised groups. Robust oversight mechanisms and practical ethical guidelines are essential to mitigate these risks.

In the United Kingdom and Europe, data sharing for health research must operate under lawful bases such as public task or legitimate interests, with appropriate safeguards. However, many individuals remain unaware that their data is being used for AI research and training. This lack of awareness can fuel distrust [15]. Meaningful transparency and early engagement with patient and public advisors can act as a safeguard, addressing these fears and fostering public trust.

Despite these challenges, patients recognise the transformative potential of AI in healthcare. Faster diagnostics, personalised treatment plans, and reduced error are among the most valued benefits. Ensuring that projects are meaningfully transparent—and surfacing and addressing fears early—is possible with the help of patient and public advisors acting as critical friends and co-designers. Patient-led governance approaches are emerging, such as The Light Collective framework [16]. Social support for sustainable change can be facilitated through patient and public advisors who help develop communications materials, but involvement can beneficially extend beyond communications development to shared decision-making across many areas of project work.

## 6.5 AI, Sustainability, and the Value of Public and Patient Participation

AI has the potential to address sustainability concerns by optimising workflows, reducing energy demands, and minimising waste [17]. Despite this promise, the environmental costs associated with AI development—such as energy-intensive model training—are gaining attention. In radiology, AI technologies offer opportunities to reduce the environmental footprint of imaging modalities like CT and MRI while improving patient care. However, impacts vary by context and require careful evaluation [17, 18].

As discussed elsewhere in this volume, green computing solutions are central to addressing sustainability in healthcare AI. These solutions demand ongoing public deliberation and value-based decisions. Claims about sustainability benefits should be evidenced and balanced against life cycle impacts. Evidence from bioethics and sustainability scholarship underscores the need for proportionate, context-specific evaluation [25].

Public involvement ensures that sustainability considerations are debated with diverse input, fostering trust in shared values and decision-making. Ongoing dialogue with public contributors supports the development of AI systems that reflect collective values, advancing patient-centred and environmentally responsible healthcare solutions.

Understanding the environmental impacts and benefits of AI is pursued in numerous projects. For example, the NetZero AICT project is conducting an environmental impact assessment involving its public advisory group to sense-check the model and build trustworthiness. This project seeks to develop sustainable and patient-centred diagnostics and reduce contrast-media-related emissions. AI-based synthetic or reduced-contrast approaches may help avoid additional scans and reduce materials use, with potential benefits for both emissions and patient safety.

Integrating AI and sustainability is not just a technological challenge but a societal one. Co-design with public contributors helps ensure that AI systems reflect shared values and priorities. A collaborative approach will help healthcare systems achieve their goals of reducing environmental impact while delivering high-quality, patient-centred care.

Public advocacy and grassroots movements further amplify calls for sustainable healthcare. For example, Flores and Samuel [19] highlight the importance of community-led initiatives in addressing the health needs of marginalised populations while advancing environmental goals. Campaigns led by the UK Health Alliance on Climate Change (UKHACC) and movements like Extinction Rebellion demonstrate the intersection of climate action, public health, and systemic reform.

Integrating patient and public perspectives into sustainability initiatives for healthcare AI not only aligns technological advancements with societal values but also builds trust and accountability.

## 6.6 Challenges and Barriers to Building Trustworthy AI Products and Projects

The integration of AI in sustainable radiology is hindered by three key challenges: lack of awareness, mistrust, and inequity. Addressing these barriers through patient and public engagement can help ensure AI innovations align with societal and environmental priorities.

Lack of Awareness and Education. Public understanding of AI's role in radiology remains limited, often obscuring its potential to enhance sustainability. Targeted, co-designed educational campaigns can clarify AI's capabilities and emphasise its role in environmentally responsible healthcare.

Mistrust and Scepticism. Concerns about data misuse, corporate motives, and opaque practices undermine trust in AI systems. Explaining how systems enhance diagnostic safety and may reduce environmental impacts, and publishing governance measures, can help to rebuild confidence.

Diverse Perspectives and Equity. Demographic disparities shape perceptions of AI and access to its benefits. Engaging diverse public contributors in design and deployment supports equity and fosters trust.

## 6.7 Strategies for Engaging Patients and the Public

Engaging patients and the public is essential for integrating AI and sustainability in radiology. Leveraging established standards and tools ensures patient and public voices shape ethical, equitable AI deployment [23]. Co-designing AI systems with public input helps address concerns like transparency, equity, and environmental impact, fostering trust and accountability.

**Education and Communication** Clear, targeted educational initiatives can bridge knowledge gaps and demystify AI's role in clinical decision-making, diagnostic accuracy, and environmental impact. The NIHR Standards for Public Involvement highlight the importance of accessible, inclusive communication. Outreach efforts such as participatory events, webinars, infographics, and collaboration with advocacy groups amplify engagement. Banerjee et al. [20] collate useful AI-engagement materials for PPIE.

**Involving Patients in Deliberation and Decision-Making** Public (and patient) advisory groups, citizens' juries, and deliberative discussions empower patients to shape AI solutions, ensuring technologies align with real-world needs and priorities. Frameworks like the NIHR's co-production guidance [2] and the Public Involvement Impact Assessment Framework [21] offer structured methodologies. Patient advisory panels can enhance confidence and quality by integrating public perspectives into governance.

**Transparency and Accountability** Transparent communication is fundamental to building trust: openly address AI benefits and risks, explain decision pathways, and publish evaluation and assurance plans.

**Tools and Resources**

- NIHR Resources and Standards for Public Involvement—https://www.learningforinvolvement.org.uk/content/resource/uk-public-involvement-standards/
- PEDRI (Patient Engagement in Data-Driven Research Initiative)—https://www.pedri.org.uk/
- EU Trustworthy AI Guidelines—https://ec.europa.eu/futurium/en/ai-alliance-consultation/guidelines/1.html
- NHS—Public Involvement Resources—https://innovation.nhs.uk/innovation-guides/development/further-information-on-ppi/

## 6.8 Conclusion

Integrating AI and sustainability in radiology offers immense potential for improving healthcare outcomes while addressing environmental challenges. However, achieving this requires a patient-centred approach prioritising trust, transparency, and inclusivity. Public involvement is recognised formally in UK policy and is embedded in European and international guidance (e.g. [8]; NIHR, 2019; [22]). As Taylor states, "Only by forming true partnerships with the public will AI in healthcare reach its full potential" [1].

Governments and regulatory bodies play a crucial role in ensuring the ethical, sustainable, and equitable use of AI in healthcare. Policies that promote green technologies, incentivise energy-efficient practice, and enforce ethical AI standards are vital. The World Health Organization emphasises human rights and ethics in the design, development, and deployment of AI for health [22].

By addressing evolving patient expectations and implementing supportive public policies, integrating AI with robust public involvement and sustainability considerations in radiology can drive innovations that are ethical, equitable, and environmentally responsible. Meaningful public engagement supports the alignment of technological advancements with societal values—ensuring that AI and sustainability initiatives are both ethical and effective. Continued collaboration between healthcare providers, technologists, policymakers, patients, and the broader public will be essential for building a future where AI enhances clinical excellence and contributes to health equity and environmental sustainability.

**Declarations**
**Funding**: Horizon 2020—NetZero AICT.

**Competing Interests**: John Kellas is stakeholder engagement lead for NetZero AICT (www.netzeroaict.eu) and director of This Equals, a UK-based public engagement consultancy company.

**Ethics Approval**: Not applicable—no studies with human participants or animals were performed by the authors for this chapter.

**Consent to Participate/Publish**: Not applicable.

**Data and/or Code Availability**: Not applicable—no new datasets or code was generated.

Parts of this chapter were drafted or edited with the assistance of generative AI tools (Perplexity, ChatGPT, and Google Gemini). The author reviewed and is responsible for the final content.

## Bibliography


1. Taylor D. AIM and the patient's perspective. In: Lidströmer N, Ashrafian H, editors. Artificial Intelligence in medicine. Cham: Springer; 2021. https://doi.org/10.1007/978-3-030-58080-3_37-1.
2. National Institute for Health Research (NIHR). Going the extra mile: improving the Nation's Health and Wellbeing through public involvement in research. London: NIHR; 2024. https://www.nihr.ac.uk/going-the-extra-mile. Accessed 15 Oct 2025
3. Medicines and Healthcare Products Regulatory Agency (MHRA), National Institute for Health and Care Research (NIHR), Health Research Authority (HRA). Public involvement in health and social care research: guidance. London: UK Government; 2022. https://www.hra.nhs.uk/planning-and-improving-research/best-practice/public-involvement/shared-commitment-public-involvement-health-and-social-care-research/. Accessed 15 Oct 2025
4. Loftus TJ, Balch JA, Abbott KL, et al. Community-engaged artificial intelligence research: a scoping review. PLOS Digit Health. 2024; https://doi.org/10.1371/journal.pdig.0000561.
5. European Environment Agency (EEA). The case for public participation in sustainability transitions. EEA Briefing 18/2023. Copenhagen: EEA; 2023. https://www.eea.europa.eu/en/analysis/publications/the-case-for-public-participation. Accessed 15 Oct 2025
6. Russell H. Public trust in AI: remarks at new statesman spotlight event. YouTube Video. 2024; https://www.youtube.com/watch?v=cfuKFtlWfTI&t=931s. Accessed 15 Oct 2025
7. Li F, Ruijs N, Lu Y. Ethics and AI: a systematic review on ethical concerns and related strategies for designing with AI in healthcare. AI. 2023;4(1):28–53. https://doi.org/10.3390/ai4010003.
8. High-Level Expert Group on AI (HLEG). Ethics guidelines for trustworthy AI. Brussels: European Commission; 2019. https://digital-strategy.ec.europa.eu/en/library/ethics-guidelines-trustworthy-ai. Accessed 15 Oct 2025

9. Blease C, O'Neill S, O'Dwyer DE, et al. Stakeholder perspectives of clinical AI implementation: systematic review of qualitative evidence. J Med Internet Res. 2023;25:e39742. https://doi.org/10.2196/39742.
10. Katirai A, Yamamoto BA, Kogetsu A, Kato K. Perspectives on Artificial Intelligence in health care from a patient and public involvement panel in Japan: an exploratory study. Front Digit Health. 2023;5:1229308. https://doi.org/10.3389/fdgth.2023.1229308.
11. The Health Foundation. AI in health care: what do the public and NHS staff think? London: The Health Foundation; 2024. https://www.health.org.uk/reports-and-analysis/analysis/ai-in-health-care-what-do-the-public-and-nhs-staff-think. Accessed 15 Oct 2025
12. Responsible Technology Adoption Unit (RTAU). Public attitudes to data and AI: tracker survey (wave 4) report. London: UK Government; 2024. https://www.gov.uk/government/publications/public-attitudes-to-data-and-ai-tracker-survey-wave-4. Accessed 15 Oct 2025
13. Hodson H. Revealed: Google AI has access to Huge Haul of NHS patient data. New Scientist. 2016; https://www.newscientist.com/article/2086454-revealed-google-ai-has-access-to-huge-haul-of-nhs-patient-data/. Accessed 15 Oct 2025
14. Royal Free London NHS Foundation Trust; DeepMind. Information Processing Agreement (IPA). (Fully Executed); 2016. https://medconfidential.org/wp-content/uploads/2016/11/DeepMind-RFL-Information-Processing-Agreement.pdf. Accessed 15 Oct 2025
15. Department of Health and Social Care (DHSC). Data saves lives: reshaping health and social care with data. London: DHSC; 2022. https://www.gov.uk/government/publications/data-saves-lives-reshaping-health-and-social-care-with-data. Accessed 15 Oct 2025
16. The Light Collective. Advocacy leaders publish first-of-its-kind governance framework—AI Rights for Patients. (Press Post, 8 Apr 2024); 2024. https://lightcollective.org/2024/04/08/advocacy-leaders-publish-first-of-its-kind-governance-framework-for-artificial-intelligence-ai-rights-for-patients/. Accessed 15 Oct 2025
17. Doo FX, Vosshenrich J, Cook TS, Moy L, Almeida EPR, Woolen SA, Gichoya JW, Heye T, Hanneman K. Environmental sustainability and AI in radiology: a double-edged sword. Radiology. 2024;310(2):e232030. https://doi.org/10.1148/radiol.232030.
18. Heye T, Merkt M, May MS, et al. The energy consumption of radiology: energy- and cost-saving opportunities for CT and MRI operation. Radiology. 2020;295(3):593–605. https://doi.org/10.1148/radiol.2020192084.
19. Flores W, Samuel J. Grassroots organisations and the right to health: are we asking the right questions? BMJ. 2019;365:l2269. https://doi.org/10.1136/bmj.l2269.
20. Banerjee S, Alsop P, Jones L, Cardinal RN. Patient and public involvement to build trust in artificial intelligence: a framework, tools, and case

studies. Patterns. 2022;3(6):100506. https://doi.org/10.1016/j.patter.2022.100506.
21. Health Data Research UK (HDR UK). PEDRI: findings from our public consultation on the Best Practice Standards for public involvement and engagement in data research and statistics. London: HDR UK; 2024. https://www.hdruk.ac.uk/wp-content/uploads/2024/05/PEDRI-Best-Practice-Standards-Report-2024.pdf. Accessed 15 Oct 2025
22. World Health Organization (WHO). Ethics and Governance of Artificial Intelligence for health. Geneva: WHO; 2021. https://www.who.int/publications/i/item/9789240029200. Accessed 15 Oct 2025
23. European Patients' Forum (EPF). AI in healthcare: advancing patient-centric care through co-design and responsible implementation. Brussels: EPF; 2023. https://www.eu-patient.eu/globalassets/policy/epf-position-paper-on-ai-in-healthcare2.pdf. Accessed 15 Oct 2025
24. Royal Free London NHS Foundation Trust. Statement regarding data processing agreement during testing of the streams app. London: Royal Free; 2016. https://www.royalfree.nhs.uk/news/statement-re-deepmind-data-processing-agreement-during-testing-phase-streams-app. Accessed 15 Oct 2025
25. Richie C (2022). Environmentally sustainable development and use of artificial intelligence in health care. Bioethics. 36(5):547–55. https://doi.org/10.1111/bioe.13018.

# Regulatory Issues in Sustainable Healthcare

# 7

Lukas Peter, Petr Straka, Aneta Kovarova, Kamil Kuca, and Petra Maresova

## 7.1 Introduction

Healthcare has become one of the most dynamically developing areas of modern society in recent decades. Technological progress, digitalization, and the pressure for efficiency have led to an unprecedented expansion of Artificial Intelligence (AI) systems into everyday clinical practice. In particular, in the field of radiology, where AI provides support in detecting abnormalities, quantifying findings, or stratifying risk, it is becoming a common part of decision-making processes.

L. Peter (✉)
Center of Advanced Innovation Technologies, VŠB-Technical University of Ostrava, Ostrava-Poruba, Czech Republic

Betthera s.r.o, Hradec Kralove, Czech Republic
e-mail: peter@betthera.com

P. Straka · A. Kovarova
Betthera s.r.o, Hradec Kralove, Czech Republic
e-mail: straka@betthera.com; kovarova@betthera.com

K. Kuca · P. Maresova
Betthera s.r.o, Hradec Kralove, Czech Republic

University of Hradec Kralove, Hradec Kralove, Czech Republic
e-mail: kuca@betthera.com; maresova@betthera.com



E. R. Ranschaert et al. (eds.), *Sustainability of AI in Radiology*, Imaging Informatics for Healthcare Professionals,
https://doi.org/10.1007/978-3-032-15693-8_7

However, as these systems expand, there is a growing need to ensure that they are not only powerful and effective but also safe, ethically acceptable, and sustainable in the long term. The answer to this challenge cannot be found only in technical development—the regulatory framework plays a key role, determining the boundaries and conditions under which new technologies are put into practice.

In this context, the concept of sustainability takes on a broader meaning. It is not only about the ecological dimension (e.g., carbon footprint or energy consumption) but also about social justice, equal access to care for patients, economic efficiency, and transparency of technological decision-making.

As WHO data shows [1, 2], the issue of sustainability of health technologies cannot be separated from fundamental infrastructural and climate challenges—more than a billion people rely on health facilities without access to electricity and sanitation.

At the same time, new concepts are emerging, such as the "regulatory genome," which represents an adaptive framework for the management and evaluation of AI systems in healthcare. The aim is to align the development of AI tools with the global sustainable development goals [3, 23, 24] and to ensure continuous oversight of their behavior in real clinical practice.

## 7.2 Current Regulatory Frameworks for AI in Healthcare

### 7.2.1 European Union

The European Union has taken an active stance toward regulating AI systems in recent years, notably through the draft proposed AI Act (formally adopted in 2024 as Regulation (EU) 2024/1689, with major obligations phased in from 2025 to 2027) and the European Health Data Space (EHDS) initiative. The AI Act is the first attempt at a horizontal legal framework that classifies AI systems according to their level of risk—from minimal to unacceptable. Systems falling into the high-risk category, which includes healthcare AI tools, are subject to strict requirements for security, transparency, traceability, documentation, and human oversight [25].

The AI Act also indirectly takes into account the level of autonomy of the system—the higher the level of autonomy, the higher the regulatory requirements for oversight, auditability, and ensuring human intervention. Systems at autonomy level 3 and above require special risk management, especially in clinical scenarios where they could replace the professional judgment of a physician [4].

As part of the EHDS initiative, the EU is working to create a harmonized environment for sharing health data between Member States, research institutions, and industry. This should support the development of AI systems with better access to training data and avoid market fragmentation.

In this context, approaches such as federated learning are also being developed, which allow training models without the need to centralize sensitive health data. This increases the protection of personal data and reduces the risk of data leakage, which is in line with the objectives of the GDPR while also strengthening sustainability in terms of cybersecurity and patient trust [5, 6, 23].

This two-tier approach—regulating AI tools themselves through the AI Act and the data environment through the EHDS—represents a fundamental shift toward the safe, interoperable, and sustainable use of AI technologies in European healthcare.

#### 7.2.1.1 AI Act a Framework for Trustworthy and Sustainable AI

The European Union Regulation on artificial intelligence (the so-called AI Act) represents the first comprehensive legislative framework aimed at regulating artificial intelligence systems across the EU. As of mid-2024, the AI Act has been formally adopted by the EU, with its provisions entering into force in 2024 and becoming fully applicable after a transition period (most high-risk requirements will apply by 2026). Early measures, like the ban on certain high-risk AI practices, take effect in 2025. The AI Act categorizes AI systems according to the level of risk (minimal, limited, high, and unacceptable) and sets out specific obligations for manufacturers, distributors, and users, in particular for so-called high-risk systems, where most medical AI applications fall.

These obligations include requirements for data quality, technical documentation, explainability, auditability, transparency, and ensuring human oversight. At the same time, the proposal repeatedly calls for the so-called sustainability by design—i.e., taking long-term sustainability into account when designing systems [23, 24].

According to some authors [4], the degree of autonomy of the system is an important aspect—higher autonomy requires more robust mechanisms for monitoring, human intervention, and risk management.

The AI Act is thus one of the key elements of the European strategy for the digital transformation of healthcare, and its implementation will be essential for the formation of a trustworthy and sustainable AI ecosystem [7].

#### 7.2.1.2 European Health Data Space (EHDS)

The EHDS is designed as a digital infrastructure and legislative framework to enable the secure sharing of health data between patients, healthcare providers, researchers, and health technology developers. This initiative [8] makes a significant contribution to the sustainable development of AI by:

- Supporting access to high-quality and interoperable data in line with the GDPR
- Enabling secondary use of data for the development, testing, and validation of AI algorithms
- Introducing requirements for cybersecurity, auditability, and governance of data spaces

For AI developers in healthcare, this means that it will be possible to test and calibrate models more efficiently in line with regulatory expectations, without violating patient privacy [9].

### 7.2.2 International Frameworks and Harmonization

The European Union plays a significant role in setting regulatory standards for medical devices using artificial intelligence, but the development of sustainable and safe AI systems in healthcare requires a globally coordinated approach. Given the nature of technologies that do not recognize geographical boundaries, it is essential that regulation is interoperable, harmonized, and based on shared principles.

The US Food and Drug Administration (FDA) has introduced the concept of the so-called Predetermined Change Control Plan (PCCP) for artificial intelligence systems that can dynamically change and learn after being launched on the market [10]. In December 2024, FDA published the final guidance "Marketing Submission Recommendations for a Predetermined Change Control Plan for Artificial Intelligence-Enabled Device Software Functions," which specifies what information manufacturers should include about planned AI model modifications, validation methods, and impact assessment within a single marketing submission. This plan allows manufacturers to define in advance the types of future updates (e.g., training with new data, changing the algorithm, adjusting the scope of use) that will be assessed and approved by the regulator during the initial assessment, thus enabling iterative improvement without the need for repeated full submissions as long as the changes stay within the pre-agreed boundaries.

This approach is also significant from a sustainability perspective—it allows for faster model iterations and reduces regulatory burden while maintaining control over the safety and functionality of the device. In practice, this means that the manufacturer does not have to repeatedly go through expensive and time-consuming approval cycles every time a minor algorithm adaptation is made [9]. The FDA also supports the use of real-world evidence (RWE) to validate the performance of models in real-world settings—i.e., data from clinical practice, which can be a key basis for decisions about further model development [11].

## 7.3 Sustainable AI: Regulatory Compliance and Life Cycle Management

Although the AI Act does not explicitly use the term "sustainability," its requirements significantly contribute to creating a framework for the development and operation of sustainable AI systems [7]. The emphasis is on transparency, robustness, security, traceability, and human oversight—aspects that not only have ethical and legal significance but also support long-term trust, stability, and effective operation of AI solutions in healthcare [24].

The Environmental, Social, Governance (ESG) framework, as described in expert analyses [12] is gradually being reflected in regulatory expectations for medical devices with AI components. These include requirements for documentation of the technology's environmental impacts, equitable access to care, inclusivity of datasets, and supply chain management. Companies are increasingly motivated to report their activities transparently through directives such as the Corporate Sustainability Reporting Directive (CSRD) and the upcoming Corporate Sustainability Due Diligence Directive (CSDDD). CSRD (Directive (EU) 2022/2464), which entered into force in January 2023, requires large EU companies and certain large non-EU companies listed on EU-regulated markets to disclose standardized sustainability information, with phased application starting from the 2024 financial year and reports to be published in 2025 and beyond. CSDDD (Directive (EU) 2024/1760), in force since July 2024, further obliges very large companies to identify and address adverse human rights and environmental impacts across their value chains. Healthcare and medtech companies that fall within the scope of these directives are therefore increasingly motivated—and in some cases legally required—to report their activities transparently [12].

AI systems must therefore be designed with sustainability by design in mind—which means not only meeting minimum requirements but also actively considering the impacts on the entire life cycle of the system, including its development, training, operation, and eventual decommissioning (i.e., the retirement of the system and its infrastructure at the end of its life cycle, in a way that minimizes waste and avoids unsupported legacy systems remaining in use). A key tool in this regard is the assessment of the carbon footprint related to computational intensity, energy consumption, and data infrastructure requirements [13].

From the perspective of long-term sustainability, it is also necessary to assess the social impacts of technologies—i.e., how they affect patients' access to healthcare and how they contribute to reducing inequalities or, conversely, risk reinforcing digital barriers. This social dimension of sustainability is increasingly considered an integral part of the technical conformity assessment and subsequent decision-making on the product's launch on the market [14].

### 7.3.1 ESG and Sustainability Principles in Regulation

In the current healthcare sector, the perception of sustainability is changing—from a topic of environmental responsibility to an integral element of regulatory and systemic policy. There is a need to understand sustainability not only as ecological but also as a structurally built-in quality of healthcare technologies, including aspects of justice, ethics, economic efficiency, and systemic management. With this shift, the ESG framework (Environmental, Social, Governance) is coming to the fore, gradually penetrating regulatory strategies in the field of medical devices, including those that use artificial intelligence.

#### 7.3.1.1 Environmental Dimension: Energy, Materials, and Ecological Footprint

The healthcare sector as a whole is a significant producer of greenhouse gas emissions—according to WHO estimates, it contributes approximately 4–5% to global emissions [2, 14]. Technology-oriented segments such as radiology or digital health further increase this impact due to high energy consumption, the need to cool data centers, and the production of electronic waste. Artificial intelligence, especially models trained by deep learning, brings significant computational demands. This phenomenon is not entirely marginal—during the training of some large language models, $CO_2$ emissions comparable to several months of operation of a mid-range car were detected [9, 15]. European regulation is starting to take these aspects into account. For example, the AI Act mentions in its preamble that artificial intelligence systems should be designed with a view to minimizing environmental impacts. This approach is referred to as "sustainable by design." In addition, the Corporate Sustainability Reporting Directive (CSRD, Directive (EU) 2022/2464), which entered into force on 5 January 2023 and is being implemented by Member States with phased application from the 2024 financial year onward, obliges large healthcare companies and other in-scope entities to report environmental indicators such as energy consumption, carbon footprint, or circularity of materials (for example, the extent to which materials and hardware used in the production and deployment of devices can be reused, repaired, or recycled within a circular economy model) [12, 16].

This approach is also linked to the increasing requirements for environmental reporting within ESG frameworks. According to analyses, the healthcare sector is among the most vulnerable in terms of ESG risks, in particular with regard to supply chain integrity, access to healthcare, and the risk of so-called greenwashing—making misleading or false claims about the technology's environmental or social benefits—when presenting technological solutions. There is growing concern that ESG compliance can become a mere box-ticking exercise; regulators and stakeholders now emphasize the need for substantive action over superficial reporting to avoid greenwashing practices.

#### 7.3.1.2 Social Dimension: Fairness, Accessibility, and Ethical Responsibility

In addition to environmental impacts, social issues also play a key role in sustainability—in particular, the accessibility of health technologies, their impartiality, and their ability to respond to the needs of different population groups. AI in healthcare is in a particularly sensitive position in this regard. Algorithms, if trained on unstructured, unbalanced, or unrepresentative data, can cause serious deviations in diagnosis, with these deviations often having the greatest impact on socially disadvantaged groups of patients.

The AI Act therefore introduces a requirement that systems falling into the high-risk category—typically those intended for diagnosis, prediction, or therapeutic decision-making—be subject to an impact assessment on fundamental human rights, including the right to fair access to healthcare [7]. The same document also requires explainability of results so that users—including patients—can make informed decisions and understand how the AI output affects their care.

From the perspective of international recommendations, it is worth noting that the WHO, in its digital health strategy, emphasizes the need for equal access to digital innovations regardless of region, social status, or language barrier [17].

#### 7.3.1.3 Governance: Accountability, Transparency, and Risk Management

Governance in the context of healthcare AI represents a framework for managing accountability, transparency, and traceability throughout the entire life cycle of the system [18]. It is closely linked to the requirements of both the Medical Device Regulation (MDR)/ In Vitro Diagnostic Regulation (IVDR) and the AI Act, but these instruments play different roles. MDR and IVDR are sector-specific product regulations focusing on the safety, performance, and clinical evidence of medical devices (including software) and specify classification rules, conformity assessment procedures, and post-market obligations. The AI Act, by contrast, is a horizontal framework that targets AI-specific risks such as data quality, opacity, robustness, and human oversight across all sectors. For AI-enabled medical devices, this means that manufacturers must design an integrated governance system that simultaneously fulfills MDR/IVDR requirements on safety and clinical performance and AI Act obligations on data, algorithms, and oversight.

A key element of governance is traceability—the ability to identify input data, the methodology used, the version of the algorithm, and the persons responsible for its development or modification. According to Goktas and Grzybowski [3], it is precisely the lack of traceability that contributes to the opacity of models and increases the risk of bias and unexplained deviations in the behavior of the system.

Sustainable AI governance also includes rules for risk management, ethical reviews, stakeholder engagement, and data access rights management. Such principles are also supported in the proposal for a European Health Data Space (EHDS), which envisages the creation of the so-called Data Access Bodies overseeing the use of AI in sensitive clinical areas.

The trustworthiness of an AI system does not come from technological quality alone, but from a combination of regulatory compliance, auditability, ethical principles, and active user involvement in the development and deployment process. Governance is thus one of the pillars of the long-term sustainability of AI in healthcare [16].

### 7.3.2 Cybersecurity and Data Protection

AI systems deployed in healthcare process a large amount of sensitive data and are therefore subject to strict requirements for cybersecurity and personal data protection. These requirements are enshrined in the European Union, primarily in the general data protection regulation (GDPR) and the network and information security directive 2 (NIS2) Directive, which complement frameworks such as the AI Act and the european health data space EHDS [2].

The NIS2 Directive (Directive on Security of Network and Information Systems) extends the obligation to manage cyber risks to key entities in the healthcare system—including healthcare service providers and manufacturers of digital medical devices. It envisages the introduction of rules for vulnerability management, mandatory incident reporting, and strengthening supplier relationships from a security perspective [12].

The General Data Protection Regulation (GDPR) plays a dual role in healthcare AI—on the one hand, it protects patient data, and on the other, it sets requirements for transparency of processing, explainability of algorithms, and consent to data processing [17]. The principles of the so-called privacy by design ensure that data collection is minimized and security measures are implemented from the beginning of the system design.

Cloud solutions and models trained outside the EU pose a particular challenge, particularly when personal health data is transmitted to jurisdictions with varying degrees of legal protection or when providers depend on nontransparent third-country infrastructures. Federated learning and decentralized methodologies provide an alternative to direct data aggregation by retaining data at its origin, yet they remain reliant on well-defined regulations for governance, interoperability, and security. The European Health Data Space (EHDS) seeks to create a framework by instituting EU-wide regulations for the main and secondary utilization of electronic health data, standardized technological specifications, and a governance framework for transnational data access. EU healthcare providers utilizing AI solutions from third countries, such as a CE-marked AI tool from Turkey, can leverage the EHDS as a “data backbone” to facilitate training, validation, and monitoring on European datasets in compliance with EU regulations while minimizing unnecessary outbound data transfers and ensuring alignment with GDPR and sector-specific legislation [5, 6, 13].

### 7.3.3 Life Cycle Management of AI Systems

Life cycle management of healthcare AI systems is a key prerequisite for their safety, quality, and long-term sustainability. This process includes design, development, validation, market launch, post-market surveillance, and system decommissioning.

#### 7.3.3.1 Algorithm Updates and Change Management

Healthcare AI systems are not static—they are subject to updates of data, models, and user interfaces. Both the MDR and the AI Act require the implementation of formal change management processes that include impact assessment, documentation of the change, and ensuring consistency with the original certification [7].

A change in the training dataset or distribution platform may affect the predictive capabilities of the system and require a reassessment of clinical validation [5, 13].

#### 7.3.3.2 Data Transparency and Traceability

The long-term credibility of AI depends on the ability to trace the origin, quality, and version of the data on which the system was trained [3]. This requirement is supported by the principles of both the GDPR and the AI Act. Traceability includes documentation of access rights, data structure, metadata, and changes in data architecture.

Without clear data documentation, validation and replicability of outputs cannot be ensured, which is an obstacle to clinical safety and regulatory sustainability [9].

#### 7.3.3.3 Performance Stability and Adaptive Systems

Sustainable systems must be able to adapt to new conditions—such as population changes, new diagnostic approaches, or technology platforms—without loss of performance or safety [19]. This requires the introduction of metrics to monitor so-called model drift and regular reassessment of predictive effectiveness.

The chapter states that without stable performance management, even a well-trained model can lose clinical value within a few months due to changes in the data.

#### 7.3.3.4 Post-Market Monitoring as Part of the Life Cycle

In the context of sustainability, two areas play a key role: post-market surveillance (PMS) and post-market clinical follow-up (PMCF). These processes ensure the ongoing monitoring of the performance of a device after its launch and are a tool for the continuous improvement of the safety, quality, and relevance of the medical device in a real clinical setting [11].

Post-market surveillance (PMS) and post-market clinical follow-up (PMCF) serve as both regulatory requirements and instruments for enduring sustainability. PMS denotes the ongoing and methodical gathering, analysis, and interpretation of data regarding the performance and safety of a device post-market release, utilizing all accessible sources. PMCF is a targeted, proactive clinical endeavor within PMS designed to address outstanding inquiries regarding clinical efficacy and residual dangers in actual usage. Collectively, they facilitate the early identification of alterations in the system's performance, behavior, or risk profile. AI manufacturers are required to establish an infrastructure for the collection of real-world data, its analysis, and the reporting of essential findings through Periodic Safety Update Reports (PSURs) for higher-risk devices, which periodically summarize the benefit-risk balance, signal detection, and any corrective or preventive measures.

In published studies [20, 21], the ability to iteratively improve based on real-world data is one of the pillars of ESG responsibility.

## 7.4 Regulatory Barriers and Opportunities for Sustainable Design

### 7.4.1 Main Barriers

Healthcare is an industry with one of the most stringent regulatory architectures ever. This framework is essential—it ensures patient safety, quality of care, and trustworthiness of systems. However, with the advent of dynamic technologies such as artificial intelligence and with the increasing emphasis on environmental and social responsibility, the structural limits of current regulatory approaches are becoming apparent, which can in some cases be counterproductive to sustainable development [22].

#### 7.4.1.1 Complexity and Cost of Compliance as a Barrier to Innovation

One of the main barriers is the high administrative and economic burden associated with achieving regulatory compliance, especially under the MDR and the AI Act [7]. For developers of AI systems, this means the need to invest significant resources in documentation, audits, clinical evaluation, cybersecurity measures, and post-market strategies. Although these requirements provide important safeguards, they often lead to a slowdown in development or the complete halt of projects with smaller budgets, especially in academic and start-up environments.

In practice, it has been repeatedly confirmed that small- and medium-sized enterprises, which are often the source of technological innovation, have limited capacities to meet all regulatory expectations. This leads either to delayed market entry or to the decision not to continue development—even in cases where the solution could have significant benefits for patients or the system as a whole [9, 16].

#### 7.4.1.2 ESG Standards and Regulatory Sustainability

Environmental, Social, and Governance (ESG) principles are becoming an integral part of the assessment of health technologies and their impact on society. While previously these factors were largely the domain of corporate voluntary reporting, current European regulations—including the Corporate Sustainability Reporting Directive (CSRD)—are putting pressure on transparent ESG reporting across sectors, including healthcare.

In conjunction with the *Corporate Sustainability Due Diligence Directive (CSDDD)*—adopted in 2024—medical device manufacturers will be required to conduct due diligence and report not only financial but also nonfinancial performance indicators, including impacts on climate, human rights, and data ethics.

These requirements directly affect the way AI systems are designed, manufactured, and monitored—for example, by focusing on the carbon footprint of the algorithm, the energy intensity of computing processes, or fair access to data and services. At the same time, there is a need to align ESG reporting with the technical documentation required by the MDR/IVDR.

#### 7.4.1.3 Flexibility and Adaptability of Regulatory Systems

Traditional regulatory frameworks such as the MDR or FDA 510(k) were designed for static products—not for AI systems that can change continuously. This poses a challenge to ensure the sustainability of these systems without compromising safety and legal certainty.

In response, new approaches are emerging, such as Principled AI or Predetermined Change Control Plan (PCCP), which allows for a predefined range of permissible changes without the need for recertification. This approach, supported by the FDA, allows manufacturers to innovate within the limits set by the regulatory plan while maintaining traceability and compliance.

European legislation has not yet formally introduced a similar tool, but the AI Act and the MDR together create space for the future adoption of similar models that will allow adaptive systems to be managed in a sustainable manner [9, 19].

#### 7.4.1.4 Ethical and Legal Uncertainty Around Decision-Making Autonomy

AI systems in clinical settings often enter an area where it can be difficult to draw a clear line between decision support and replacement of medical judgment. Current regulatory frameworks require the presence of human oversight, but practice shows that as AI becomes more reliable, its outputs can be interpreted as de facto authoritative. Regulation does not yet provide detailed guidance on how to address liability for errors caused by "soft suggestion" systems, which creates uncertainty for both developers and users [2]. However, the EU has recently moved to address part of this gap: a revised Product Liability Directive was adopted in late 2024, extending liability to software and AI systems and easing the burden of proof for injured parties. This will make it easier for patients to seek compensation for harm caused by defective AI tools, although clear guidance on apportioning responsibility between clinicians and AI systems remains undeveloped.

This uncertainty often leads to a defensive stance by institutions that are afraid to deploy AI solutions despite their potential benefits—creating the paradox of regulation as a tool that hinders positive systemic change rather than protecting it.

### 7.4.2 Opportunities When Regulations Support Sustainable Design

While regulation can be seen as a limiting factor, in the area of sustainability, AI in healthcare is also an important tool for supporting environmentally and socially responsible approaches. Well-established regulatory frameworks create space for innovations that would not be economically feasible or sufficiently trustworthy under normal market conditions.

In several strategic documents, the WHO recommends the integration of AI systems into broader concepts of so-called green hospitals (climate-smart healthcare), which include energy efficiency, waste management, safe handling of chemicals, and operational optimization. In this context, AI can be used not only as a diagnostic tool but also as a predictive system for managing logistics, energy consumption, or care planning [17].

A specific framework for assessing the environmental maturity of AI solutions is also offered by the so-called ESG maturity model [20], which distinguishes three levels of approach: basic (compliance-driven), normative (standard-based), and eco-social (value-integrated). This model can be useful not only for developers but also for evaluators in the certification process.

It can also be mentioned that regulations that enable adaptive management (e.g., through PMS and PMCF) allow systems to respond flexibly to environmental changes, thereby increasing their long-term efficiency and environmental friendliness. This is in line with the concept of so-called adaptive healthcare, which emphasizes continuous learning and adjustment of care pathways based on real-world data and feedback from practice [14].

Regulation can thus become an engine for a positive transformation of healthcare toward greater sustainability—not only from an environmental perspective but also from an economic and social perspective. It promotes reuse, reduces regulatory uncertainty, and creates trust in new technologies among care providers, patients, and payers of the system.

#### 7.4.2.1 Life Cycle Support as a Framework for Continuous Optimization

The MDR requirements for PMS and PMCF create a framework for long-term monitoring and improvement of the performance of AI systems [11]. This framework allows for continuous performance evaluation without the need for recertification, thereby supporting:

- Extension of the life of devices (reducing the need to replace them with new ones)
- Software modularity, which allows for partial updates without interfering with the entire system
- Accumulation of knowledge leading to more efficient and less demanding algorithms

This makes the regulatory framework a tool for a circular approach to innovation—manufacturers are motivated to optimize existing products instead of developing completely new generations [23].

#### 7.4.2.2 ESG and Nonfinancial Reporting as a Bridge Between Regulation and Strategy

The Corporate Sustainability Reporting Directive (CSRD) and the draft Corporate Sustainability Due Diligence Directive (CSDDD) oblige companies to report ESG indicators, including environmental impact, social approaches, and governance structures [22]. These requirements are not primarily medical, but are increasingly being included in the regulation of medical devices and in the requirements for manufacturers.

As shown by the Clifford Chance analysis, it is precisely the connection of ESG teams with legal and compliance departments that can reveal previously unaddressed opportunities—for example:

- Optimization of medical device packaging
- Shortening the supply chain (and thus reducing the carbon footprint)
- Introducing ethical standards for the use of data, especially in global projects with the risk of modern slavery or violation of patient rights (ESG and compliance)

These initiatives are not based on the MDR or AI Act, but they are complementary to them—well-maintained technical documentation allows for easy integration of ESG considerations into internal quality management system (QMS) processes, thereby creating synergy between regulatory compliance and corporate strategy [24].

#### 7.4.2.3 Harmonization as a Means of Reducing Costs and Promoting Sustainability

Different jurisdictions often approach the regulation of medical devices differently, which increases the duplicative burden for manufacturers and complicates the implementation of sustainable solutions. However, initiatives such as the International Medical Device Regulators Forum (IMDRF) [18] are working to unify basic requirements, which can lead to:

- Reducing the number of necessary audits and recertifications
- Unifying data interoperability requirements, which allows for easier transfer of AI models between markets
- Faster replication of successful solutions in different regions

All this leads to a reduction in environmental burden and regulatory costs, and therefore to a more efficient use of resources while maintaining a high level of patient safety [23].

## 7.5 Regulatory Recommendations and Strategic Directions for Sustainable AI

Promoting sustainability in healthcare AI does not only result from technological innovation but also requires active and targeted regulatory interventions. Well-designed regulatory frameworks can serve as accelerators for the transition to climate-responsible, socially just, and long-term functional systems.

A useful framework for assessing the level of integration of sustainability into the development of healthcare AI tools is the so-called ESG maturity model [20]. It distinguishes three approaches: compliance-driven, where the organization only fulfills the necessary legislative obligations; normative (standards-based), where it relies on established industry standards; and the highest level of eco-social (value-integrated), where sustainability is part of the company's mission and values.

Numerous research teams and industry coalitions have lately commenced investigations on "sustainability scores" or labels for digital health technologies and AI systems, intending to furnish transparent and comparable data regarding their environmental and social performance. None of these initiatives has yet evolved into a broadly accepted or compulsory framework; however, they exemplify a potential future where ESG-related measurements may attain visibility comparable to conventional safety and performance indicators for consumers and regulators. Simultaneously, experts caution that inadequately structured scoring systems may facilitate greenwashing by emphasizing easily quantifiable indicators while neglecting more profound structural difficulties, such as supply chain implications or rebound phenomena.

Special attention should be paid to post-market surveillance (PMS) and post-market clinical follow-up (PMCF), which can play a crucial role in managing sustainability in a real-world environment. This data not only helps monitor system performance and risks but also allows identifying room for improvement in terms of environmental efficiency or social impact [24].

Last but not least, it is important that regulatory frameworks support small- and medium-sized enterprises, which often come up with innovative and sustainable solutions but face disproportionate certification costs. Simplified pathways, pre-populated templates, or shared reference datasets (as proposed by the EHDS) can be important tools on the path to greater accessibility and scale-up of sustainable AI.

### 7.5.1 Integrating ESG Indicators into Technical Documentation

With the increasing emphasis on the social responsibility of health technologies, it is desirable that ESG reporting is not a separate corporate agenda, but an integral part of the technical documentation and quality management system of medical devices.

We recommend that regulatory frameworks—for example, through updates to the MDR annexes or the MDCG methodological guidelines—allow manufacturers to include selected ESG indicators in the conformity assessment [12, 22]. Suitable indicators include, for example:

- Carbon footprint of the algorithm and its training
- Method of data acquisition and preprocessing (including bias)
- Methods for reducing the energy intensity of operation
- Measures for the social accessibility of the system (language, digital literacy)
- Quality of communication with the patient and ethics of the outputs

Such a structured integration of ESG into the approval processes will allow both greater transparency and a proactive approach to sustainability on the part of manufacturers. At the same time, harmonizing the requirements with the CSRD/CSDDD will reduce the administrative burden and strengthen the trust of all stakeholders [20].

### 7.5.2 Expansion of Adaptive Regulatory Models

A fundamental obstacle to long-term sustainability is the current concept of changes and updates in European regulation, which continues to be based on a static paradigm. However, AI systems are inherently dynamic—they adapt to new data, update models, and change their decision-making strategies. The FDA's approach through the Predetermined Change Control Plan (PCCP) can be an inspiration; it defines a framework of permissible future changes that have been previously regulatory approved and do not require reassessment Protocol for Iterative Improvement and Sustainability (PIIS).

Introducing a similar mechanism within the MDR or AI Act would allow:

- Flexible management of updates without the need for complete recertification,
- Faster adaptation of systems to new clinical findings
- Reduced environmental impacts associated with HW replacement or development of completely new versions

Manufacturers could thus plan a longer-term system life cycle without worrying about regulatory complications with each technical modification.

### 7.5.3 Standardization, Harmonization as a Tool for Sustainability

The lack of data standardization and incompatibility between systems increases costs, burdens the infrastructure, and complicates the development of sustainable models. Regulation should explicitly support the use of open data formats and frameworks (e.g., Health Level Seven (HL7), Fast Healthcare Interoperability Resources (FHIR), Digital Imaging and Communications in Medicine (DICOM), Observational Medical Outcomes Partnership (OMOP), Common Data Model (CDM)) and incentivize manufacturers to develop systems with a high level of interoperability [24].

International cooperation is not just a matter of regulatory convenience. It is essential for the sustainability of technology development and implementation. Harmonization enables:

- Shortening the development and market launch time thanks to shared assessment frameworks
- Reducing the administrative and documentation burden, which has a direct impact on the consumption of material and human resources
- Greater transparency of data requirements, which supports data reuse and optimization of computational processes
- Better portability of technologies to different healthcare systems, including those with limited capacities

From the perspective of the ESG framework, harmonization is a path to efficient use of resources, reducing barriers to access for patients across regions and strengthening accountability in the management of global healthcare innovations. However, to achieve these goals, harmonization must not only be technical but also include shared values—especially in the areas of ethics, social justice, and environmental responsibility [25].

## 7.6 Conclusion

The development of artificial intelligence in healthcare, and in particular in the field of radiology, represents an unprecedented opportunity to increase the efficiency, accessibility, and quality of healthcare. However, with this potential come new regulatory challenges that require legal frameworks to reflect not only technical safety and performance but also the broader impacts of these technologies on society and the environment. This chapter has shown that regulatory approaches play a crucial role not only in protecting patients but also in defining the direction of healthcare innovation and in supporting or blocking sustainable development.

Based on the analysis of current European and international regulations—including the MDR, AI Act, GDPR, NIS2, and EHDS—it can be stated that regulation is starting to naturally expand toward greater transparency, accountability, and sustainability. However, there is still a lack of clear and structured integration of ESG criteria into technical documentation, assessment frameworks, and strategic decision-making. Regulations still primarily assess safety and performance, not the environmental footprint, the circular nature of the system, or social equality in access to technologies.

Special attention was paid to the life cycle management of AI systems, which is essential not only from the point of view of safety but also from the point of view of long-term relevance and resource efficiency. Mechanisms such as PMS and PMCF are not just compliance tools—they become active quality management and accountability tools. Strengthening them with nonfinancial indicators could bring a new standard for documenting the sustainable operation of healthcare AI.

International cooperation also plays a crucial role. Fragmentation of regulatory approaches between the USA, EU, and other jurisdictions represents not only an economic burden but also an environmental inefficiency. Global harmonization of procedures, sharing of audit frameworks, and open standardization of data structures are a condition for AI to be truly scalable and sustainable in the long term.

The aim of regulatory policy should therefore be not only to prevent harm but also to actively support technologies that bring systemic improvements to healthcare. This includes not only classic compliance but also supporting tools such as predefined change frameworks, regulatory sandboxes, ESG reporting, and support for academic teams. Without this support, sustainable AI may be doomed to marginality—despite its potential.

This chapter shows that regulation and sustainability are not opposites, but two sides of the same coin. Responsible regulation is a prerequisite for the credibility, quality, and social acceptability of artificial intelligence. And in the field of healthcare, where human life is the highest value, these principles must be consistently linked.

## Bibliography


1. Canton H. World Health Organization—WHO. In: The Europa directory of international organizations 2021. Routledge; 2021. p. 370–84.
2. Guidance WHO. Ethics and governance of artificial intelligence for health. World Health Organization; 2021.
3. Goktas P, Grzybowski A. Shaping the future of healthcare: ethical clinical challenges and pathways to trustworthy AI. J Clin Med. 2025;14(5):1605.
4. Bitterman DS, Aerts HJWL, Mak RH. Approaching autonomy in medical artificial intelligence. Lancet Digital Health. 2020;2(9):e447–9.
5. Long G, et al. Federated learning for privacy-preserving open innovation future on digital health. In: Humanity driven AI: productivity, well-being, sustainability and partnership. Cham: Springer; 2021. p. 113–33.
6. Kanter GP, Packel EA. Health care privacy risks of AI Chatbots. JAMA. 2023;330(4):311–2.

7. Cantero Gamito M, Marsden CT. Artificial intelligence co-regulation? The role of standards in the EU AI Act. Int J Law Inf Technol. 2024;32(1):eaae011.
8. Marcus JS, et al. The European health data space. IPOL| Policy Department for Economic, Scientific and Quality of Life Policies, European Parliament Policy Department Studies; 2022.
9. Marešová P, et al. Complexity stage model of the medical device development based on economic evaluation – MedDee. Sustainability. 2020;12(5):1755.
10. Intelligence, FDA Artificial. Machine Learning in Software as a Medical Device Action Plan. 2021 [online].
11. Process, Clearance. Medical devices and the public's health: the FDA 510 (k) clearance process at 35 years. Washington, DC: Institute of Medicine of the National Academies; 2011.
12. Leung TCH, You CS-X. ESG application in sustainable development of the healthcare industry. In: Environmental, social and governance and sustainable development in healthcare. Singapore: Springer; 2023. p. 47–64.
13. Folland S, et al. The economics of health and health care. Routledge; 2024.
14. Caltagirone A, et al. From regulations to strategy for sustainable healthcare by 2030. J Prev Med Hyg. 2025;65(4):E476.
15. Chen Z. ESG practice of medical device companies and its impact on corporate performance: taking mindray as an example. In: SHS web of conferences. EDP sciences; 2024. p. 01013.
16. Bouderhem R. Ethical and regulatory challenges for AI biosensors in healthcare. In: Proceedings. MDPI; 2024. p. 37.
17. World Health Organization. A global health strategy for 2025–2028-advancing equity and resilience in a turbulent world: fourteenth general programme of work. World Health Organization; 2025.
18. Fraser AG, et al. Artificial intelligence in medical device software and high-risk medical devices–a review of definitions, expert recommendations and regulatory initiatives. Expert Rev Med Devices. 2023;20(6):467–91.
19. OCL H, Burnham KJ, editors. Intelligent and adaptive systems in medicine. CRC Press; 2008.
20. Farah L, et al. Suitability of the current health technology assessment of innovative artificial intelligence-based medical devices: scoping literature review. J Med Internet Res. 2024;26:e51514.
21. Chen R, Zhang T. Artificial intelligence applications implication for ESG performance: can digital transformation of enterprises promote sustainable development? Chin Manag Stud. 2024;
22. Candio P, et al. Sustainability and corporate performance in health care. Springer; 2024.

23. Romagnoli A, et al. Healthcare systems and artificial intelligence: focus on challenges and the international regulatory framework. Pharm Res. 2024;41(4):721–30.
24. Pantanowitz L, et al. Regulatory aspects of AI-ML. Mod Pathol. 2024:100609.
25. Ukhova D, et al. Public health approaches to gambling: a global review of legislative trends. Lancet Public Health. 2024;9(1):e57–67.

# 8 Toward a Sustainable Future of AI in Healthcare Imaging

Saif Afat, Judith Herrmann, and Thomas Küstner

## 8.1 Introduction

Artificial intelligence (AI) has rapidly transformed healthcare, delivering notable gains in diagnostic accuracy, operational efficiency, and patient outcomes. In medical imaging, spanning diagnostic radiology, radiation therapy, interventional radiology, and nuclear medicine, AI adoption is particularly advanced, with many AI-powered devices already cleared for clinical use. These applications streamline workflows, improve image interpretation, shorten examination times, and reduce reliance on contrast agents. Such improvements not only enhance patient comfort but also improve access to care by reducing the need for unnecessary

S. Afat · J. Herrmann
Department of Diagnostic and Interventional Radiology, University Hospital Tübingen, Tübingen, Germany
e-mail: saif.afat@med.uni-tuebingen.de; judith.herrmann@med.uni-tuebingen.de

T. Küstner (✉)
Medical Image and Data Analysis (MIDAS.lab), Department of Diagnostic and Interventional Radiology, University Hospital Tübingen, Tübingen, Germany

Institute for Bioinformatics and Medical Informatics, Eberhard-Karls University of Tuebingen, Tuebingen, Germany
e-mail: thomas.kuestner@med.uni-tuebingen.de



E. R. Ranschaert et al. (eds.), *Sustainability of AI in Radiology*, Imaging Informatics for Healthcare Professionals,
https://doi.org/10.1007/978-3-032-15693-8_8

travel for patients and staff. Some analyses even project that autonomous AI systems could reduce healthcare-related greenhouse gas (GHG) emissions by up to 80% [1].

Yet, this promise comes with a cost: AI is among the most resource-intensive digital technologies, requiring substantial computational power for model training, deployment, and maintenance—activities that carry significant energy and water demands. Training a single large-scale model can emit more than 626,000 pounds of $CO_2$ (≈313 t), equivalent to the lifetime emissions of several gasoline-powered cars [2]. Even smaller models deployed on cloud-based infrastructure contribute to both energy consumption and water usage. AI's infrastructure and, in particular, cloud-based data centers already consume more electricity than some industrial sectors and use vast volumes of water for cooling [3, 4]. Globally, emissions from data storage alone are now estimated to exceed those of the entire aviation industry. Historically, these environmental costs have been largely overlooked in discussions concerning the role of AI in healthcare.

Medical imaging amplifies this tension. Healthcare as a whole contributes about 4.6% of global GHG emissions, and imaging accounts for roughly 10% of the sector's footprint, which is equivalent to about 1% of total global $CO_2$ emissions [5]. Magnetic resonance imaging (MRI) and CT dominate this share due to their high electricity consumption, large data outputs, reliance on contrast media, and associated waste. A single MRI scanner consumes, on average, more than 100 MWh annually, making it the most energy-intensive device in radiology [6, 7]. Even in "system-off" mode, MRI units consume 31–38% of their annual energy (35–47 MWh) to maintain magnet superconductivity, and over half of all scanners worldwide remain powered at full idle during nonproductive hours. CT scanners, while less energy-intensive than MRI, still draw 20,000–35,000 kWh per year [7]. Contrast agents such as iodinated compounds and gadolinium-based chelates are another environmental concern: an estimated 19 tons of gadolinium enter EU wastewater annually (21 tons in the US) [8], and ultrasound contrast agents containing sulfur hexafluoride ($SF_6$) carry a 100-year global warming potential of 25,200 kg $CO_2$ e per kilogram released [9].

As AI becomes increasingly integrated into the domain of precision medicine, the demand for even larger datasets and more complex algorithms is set to rise—escalating energy consumption and associated environmental impacts. This chapter critically examines this "double-edged sword" [9]: AI holds promise for improving the sustainability of medical imaging through efficiency gains and resource optimization; it simultaneously contributes to the healthcare sector's carbon footprint. The aim is to explore practical strategies for minimizing AI's environmental costs while preserving, and ideally enhancing, its clinical benefits.

## 8.2 The Environmental Footprint of Medical Imaging and AI

The healthcare sector is a major GHG emitter, responsible for around 4.6% of total global emissions [5]. In 2009, the US health system alone accounted for 8.5% of national emissions, a proportion that increased by 6% between 2010 and 2018 [10]. On a global scale, if the Chinese and American healthcare systems were treated as independent nations, they would rank as the 10th and 14th largest carbon emitters, respectively. Hospitals are disproportionately large contributors, producing roughly 35% of the sector's total emissions.

Within healthcare, medical imaging, including diagnostic and interventional radiology, accounts for an estimated 10% of emissions. Diagnostic imaging alone represents about 1% of the total global $CO_2$ footprint. This impact arises primarily from the high energy requirements of MRI and CT, the production and disposal of contrast agents, data storage demands, and patient and staff transportation [5].

### 8.2.1 Baseline Environmental Impact by Modality

**Magnetic Resonance Imaging (MRI)**

MRI is among the most energy-intensive modalities due to its reliance on superconducting magnets and continuous cooling systems. Annual consumption for a modern MRI unit ranges from 80,000 to 170,000 kWh, comparable to the yearly use of 16–34 four-person households in Germany [6, 7]. Even when idle, an MRI consumes 7–9 kW to maintain magnet temperature via helium cooling, representing 31–38% of total annual energy use [6] with idle/standby periods representing 50–60% of total usage time [11, 12]. This waste is further magnified by the fact that over half of MRI scanners worldwide are never powered down outside clinical hours. Cooling the gradient coils, which are capable of reaching >60 °C during operation, requires additional closed-loop heat exchange systems. Manufacturing is also energy-intensive: producing a single MRI system consumes about 2.73 million MJ (~753,000 kWh) of fossil fuel energy, equivalent to the annual emissions of 73 gasoline-powered cars [13].

**Computed Tomography (CT)**

CT scanners consume 20,000–35,000 kWh annually, equal to 4–7 four-person households in Germany [7]. In one university hospital study, the combined annual electricity use of three CT and four MRI scanners plus cooling exceeded 1.1 million kWh, about 4% of total hospital consumption, comparable to the needs of a town of 852 people [7]. Each CT scan produces roughly 6.6 kg $CO_2$e, with energy drawn primarily during gantry operation.

**Positron Emission Tomography (PET)**

PET/CT imaging has a substantial carbon footprint; one study estimated around 2.01 kg $CO_2$ e per PET/CT procedure, with the scanner's electricity consumption contributing approximately 62% of that total [14]. Beyond electricity, PET carries environmental costs from the production, transport, and disposal of radiotracers. These processes involve radioactive materials and generate hazardous waste. In some life cycle assessments, PET's overall footprint has been found to rival or surpass that of cardiac MRI protocols [15].

**Ultrasound (US)**

Ultrasound is the least energy- and carbon-intensive modality. A single abdominal ultrasound produces ~0.5 kg $CO_2$ e which is more than 10 times less than CT and over 30 times less than MRI [16]. Annual consumption for a modern US system is ~2500 kWh, about half the electricity and $CO_2$ output of one four-person household in Europe.

### 8.2.2 Additional Environmental Burdens from AI Integration

The environmental footprint of medical imaging increases when AI is layered onto baseline operations. While the energy demands of model training are well recognized, large-scale inference also incurs significant energy costs. Deploying AI across extensive hospital networks or cloud-based platforms, especially for real-time or high-throughput applications, can require substantial computational resources, raising critical questions about the sustainability of such systems.

**Model Training and Inference**
Training large AI models is highly energy-intensive. A single large-scale training run can emit as much $CO_2$ as five cars over their entire lifespan [2]. Training emissions for a language model on the scale of GPT-3 have been estimated between 223,920 and 858,360 kg $CO_2$ e, depending on infrastructure and energy source—equivalent to the annual emissions of 50–191 passenger cars [17]. Although each inference (model prediction) consumes far less energy than training, frequent use scales rapidly. In medical imaging, models may not reach the scale of current large language models (GPT, Claude, Grok, Gemini), but cumulative impacts still add up when numerous specialized networks are run for different modalities, organs, and clinical tasks. In high-volume clinical environments, cumulative inference emissions are even estimated to surpass training emissions [2].

**Data Centers and Cooling**
Data centers consume 1–2% of global electricity, with total cloud-storage emissions now estimated to exceed those of aviation [3]. Data centers also have large water footprints: globally, they con-

sume around 626 billion gallons per year for cooling and power generation. Projected AI growth could raise this to 4.2–6.6 billion $m^3$ by 2027—more than half the UK's annual water use [4]. Carbon intensity depends heavily on local energy mix; shifting workloads to renewable-powered regions can yield large reductions.

**Resource Extraction and e-Waste**
Manufacturing GPUs, CPUs, and other high-performance computing components relies on energy-intensive mining of rare earths and metals like cobalt, lithium, and tantalum, often with environmental and social harms [18]. Without effective refurbishment and recycling programs, retired hardware adds to electronic waste burdens.

### 8.2.3 Life Cycle Analysis in Imaging AI

Life cycle analysis (LCA) quantifies environmental impacts from raw material extraction through manufacturing, operation, and end-of-life disposal. The healthcare sector generates significant e-waste when imaging systems and supporting hardware are decommissioned. Without effective refurbishment and recycling programs, valuable materials are lost, and hazardous waste can enter the environment. For MRI, the production phase alone consumes ~2.73 million MJ of fossil fuels (~753,000 kWh), producing GHG emissions equivalent to a year's driving for 73 cars [13]. Ultrasound consistently shows the lowest life cycle footprint, while MRI ranks highest.

Applying LCA to AI in imaging is essential for understanding the full environmental cost of model development, deployment, hardware use, and downstream consequences of disposal. Investigations need to be carried out to identify opportunities to reduce impact at each stage. Recognizing these costs is the first step toward designing strategies that mitigate them while preserving the clinical benefits of AI.

## 8.3 AI for Sustainable Medical Imaging: Opportunities and Strategies

AI offers multiple pathways to improve the environmental sustainability of medical imaging. These range from optimizing workflows and reducing unnecessary examinations to shortening scan times, lowering reliance on high-impact consumables, and enabling alternative diagnostic strategies. Importantly, many of these benefits are no longer just theoretical. Practical implementations already demonstrate measurable impact. At the same time, reducing the environmental footprint of AI itself requires efficient algorithms, careful hardware selection, sustainable data management, and life cycle-conscious infrastructure planning [9]. Together, these approaches form a dual strategy: using AI to make imaging greener while making AI itself greener.

### 8.3.1 Workflow Optimization and Reduction of Low-Value Imaging

Approximately 20–50% of medical imaging tests are classified as low value—providing little or no clinical benefit while consuming energy and resources [19–25]. AI-enabled clinical decision support tools can help target and reduce this unnecessary activity by providing personalized, evidence-based imaging recommendations at the point of order [26, 27].

Beyond optimizing ordering, AI can streamline the operational flow of imaging services. Intelligent scheduling algorithms can analyze historical appointment patterns, predict peak demand, and identify patients likely to miss appointments. This enables departments to reallocate slots in real time, reduce scanner idle periods, and coordinate multiple examinations within a single visit. By minimizing unproductive machine time and unnecessary patient travel, such tools have the potential to directly reduce associated GHG emissions.

In theory, AI could also monitor scanner activity and predict idle intervals for MRI and CT systems, triggering automated power-downs during nonclinical hours and energy-efficient reactivation before the next scheduled patient. Similar predictive approaches could extend to peripheral systems, such as PACS workstations, to reduce idle energy draw.

### 8.3.2 Accelerated Acquisition and Energy Savings

Scan duration is directly proportional to the active energy consumption of MRI systems, making acquisition speed a critical determinant of environmental impact. AI-based reconstruction methods enable the acquisition of highly undersampled data and thereby shorten MRI protocols without sacrificing diagnostic quality.

Evidence from musculoskeletal MRI demonstrates that AI-accelerated sequences can reduce scan times by up to 71% and energy use by 72% compared with conventional protocols. On an annual basis, this translates into savings of approximately 14.1 MWh per scanner—equivalent to 5422 kg $CO_2$ in Germany [6]. Across a practice performing 24 MRI examinations per day, 7 days per week, accelerating protocols by 25–75% was projected to save 200.6–867.1 MWh annually and avoid 140.2–606.1 t $CO_2$ e; these projections were derived from 377 clinical examinations logged across three MRI scanners [28].

While AI reconstruction requires additional computation, the energy savings from reduced acquisition time generally outweigh the reconstruction cost. Moreover, faster protocols increase scanner throughput, reducing the need for additional MRI units and thus avoiding the energy and manufacturing footprint of new hardware.

Beyond acceleration [29, 30], AI supports sustainability through automated plane planning, which shortens setup time [31, 32], and cross-modality synthesis, such as generating CT-equivalent images from MRI [33, 34], which avoids the need for additional scans. AI is also being used to enhance images from lower-field MRI systems, enabling the use of more energy-efficient scanners [35–37]. In parallel, AI-driven triage tools can automatically identify urgent or high-priority cases on imaging worklists, accelerating diagnosis for time-critical conditions such as acute pulmonary embolism. Importantly, these systems can also be designed with operational and environmental efficiency in mind, for example, by grouping cases to optimize scanner scheduling or aligning imaging appointments with other outpatient visits to reduce patient travel [16].

### 8.3.3 Dose Optimization and Contrast Reduction

AI can optimize CT and PET protocols to reduce radiation dose without compromising image quality. In CT, algorithms can automatically refine patient positioning, adjust tube current, and reconstruct diagnostic-quality images from lower-dose data. For PET, AI-enhanced reconstruction enables shorter acquisition times or reduced tracer doses, lessening both patient exposure and radiopharmaceutical production needs.

A major environmental benefit of AI lies in reducing contrast media use. Gadolinium-based agents, used in MRI, and iodinated agents, used in CT, are both environmentally persistent and have measurable ecological impact. AI-powered imaging sequences can either improve image quality at reduced contrast doses or generate synthetic contrast-enhanced images from low-dose or even non-contrast datasets. In CT, such approaches can cut iodinated contrast usage by up to 50% [38]. In MRI, deep-learning-based virtual native enhancement techniques can delineate ischemic or fibrotic myocardial tissue with results comparable to standard contrast-enhanced scans, reducing gadolinium consumption [9].

### 8.3.4 Remote and Decentralized Diagnostics

By enabling remote image acquisition, interpretation, and consultation, the need for patient and staff travel cuts associated emissions. In teleradiology, AI can support quality assurance for images acquired at decentralized sites, allowing more cases to be handled locally rather than referred to central hospitals [39–41].

Point-of-care US offers an especially low-carbon diagnostic alternative to MRI and CT for many clinical scenarios [42] which is approximately 0.65 kg $CO_2$ e for an abdominal exam compared to 2.61 kg for CT and 13.72 kg for MRI [43–46]. AI can further increase its clinical applicability by standardizing acquisition, reducing operator variability, and improving diagnostic accuracy. Its portability also avoids transport- and hospital-related emissions [46].

### 8.3.5 Industry and Hospital Initiatives with Life Cycle Thinking

Sustainability requires action at the system level, encompassing both industry and healthcare institutions. Medical imaging vendors are beginning to adopt measures that align product design with sustainability goals. Some now publish Environmental Product Declarations (EPDs) that disclose the life cycle impacts of their equipment, while others incorporate automated energy-saving modes and design scanners for modular upgrades, allowing up to 95% reuse of components [47]. Industry-wide collaborations such as those led by the European Coordination Committee of the Radiological, Electromechanical and Healthcare IT Industry (COCIR) are working to standardize environmental performance metrics [48]. A radiology-specific eco-label, similar to the "Energy Star" program, would help purchasers compare imaging solutions not just by diagnostic performance but also by environmental impact.

A sustainable approach to AI and imaging technology must consider environmental impacts across the entire life cycle, from manufacturing to end of life. Life cycle assessment (LCA; see Sect. 8.2.3) provides a framework for evaluating this full spectrum. Designing scanners for modular upgrades rather than full replacement amplifies sustainability gains by extending equipment life and reducing the need for energy-intensive manufacturing.

At the other end of the life cycle, responsible disposal of e-waste is essential to prevent toxic materials such as lead, cadmium, and mercury from contaminating the environment. Hospitals can also reduce overall waste generation by transitioning to paperless workflows, recycling consumables, and engaging vendors in efforts to streamline packaging and encourage the return or refurbishment of parts. Regular maintenance not only prolongs equipment life but also improves energy efficiency over time [49].

At the institutional level, hospitals are embedding AI within broader sustainability strategies. Departments are appointing sustainability officers and setting measurable environmental targets [9, 47, 48]. AI-driven operational tools can predict idle scanner periods and automatically power down systems, optimize appointment scheduling to minimize patient travel, and identify opportunities to consolidate workloads to reduce equipment use [50]. Procurement policies increasingly require environmental performance assessments before acquiring new equipment, and waste reduction initiatives which range from minimizing single-use items to enhancing recycling and circular economy practices, are becoming common [51]. Education and training initiatives are equally important, ensuring that clinicians and technical staff understand how AI can contribute to sustainable imaging and how their daily decisions impact environmental outcomes [52].

### 8.3.6 Algorithmic Efficiency

The most direct way to lower AI's carbon footprint is to reduce the computational effort required for model training and inference. Techniques such as pruning [53], quantization [54], and knowledge distillation [55] can dramatically shrink model size, eliminate redundant parameters, and cut processing time without significant loss in accuracy. Pruning selectively removes unnecessary neurons and connections; quantization reduces numerical precision in model weights and activations, which accelerates inference while lowering power consumption; and distillation trains a smaller "student" model to replicate the performance of a larger "teacher" model. Transfer learning [56] also plays a critical role by fine-tuning pretrained networks for specific medical imaging tasks, avoiding the need for costly training from scratch. In some cases, probabilistic models can replace more complex deterministic ones, offering substantial energy savings when perfect accuracy is not essential. Open-source optimization frameworks have demonstrated that such approaches can reduce the energy demands of deep learning models by 15–76% [57–60]. Importantly, model development in healthcare should resist the temptation to chase marginal accuracy gains at the cost of exponentially higher computational loads, instead focusing on clinically meaningful innovation.

### 8.3.7 Hardware Optimization

Hardware choices influence energy consumption as much as model architecture. While GPUs remain the workhorse for image processing due to their parallel computing capabilities, they are also among the most energy-intensive components in AI workflows. Alternatives such as tensor processing units (TPUs) and field-programmable gate arrays (FPGAs) offer substantial efficiency gains for certain workloads [61]. Emerging paradigms, including neuromorphic and quantum computing techniques, promise even greater reductions in energy demand, though their application in medical imaging is still experimental [62–66]. Tiny machine learning (tinyML) represents another promising path by running AI models on low-power edge devices, reducing reliance on energy-hungry central servers [67]. Even modest adjustments to hardware configuration can lead to noticeable reductions in energy use and associated emissions, without major performance penalties.

### 8.3.8 Data Management

The way medical imaging data is stored and accessed has significant environmental implications. Selective long-term retention of essential image data, combined with the elimination of redundant reconstructions that can be regenerated when needed, can greatly reduce storage requirements. Compression and deduplication technologies help shrink file sizes and eliminate duplicate datasets, lowering both storage energy costs and cooling requirements. Tiered storage systems, in which frequently accessed data is kept on fast, energy-efficient media while older or rarely accessed files are archived on lower-power storage devices, provide an effective balance between accessibility and sustainability. Federated learning [68] offers an additional advantage by allowing models to be trained across multiple institutions without centralizing raw datasets, thereby reducing the emissions associated with large-scale data transfers and centralized storage [69]. Sustainability-conscious health networks are increasingly seeking cloud providers that commit to renewable energy sourcing and energy-conscious scheduling of high-load processing [70].

### 8.3.9 Greening Infrastructure

Since data centers form the operational backbone of AI in imaging, their energy and water use must be addressed directly. Powering these facilities with renewable energy sources such as wind and solar can dramatically reduce their carbon footprint, while cooling innovations like free-air, liquid, or immersion cooling can lower the electricity used for climate control, which often accounts for up to 40% of a data center's total consumption [71–73]. Water footprint monitoring is equally important, especially in regions vulnerable to scarcity. In the imaging domain, AI tools can predict idle scanner periods and automate shutdowns and restarts to minimize nonproductive energy consumption (see Sect. 8.3.2). Waste heat recovery systems can also repurpose the thermal energy generated by scanners or server rooms to warm clinical spaces, reducing the demand on separate heating systems.

In summary, AI's ability to optimize workflows, shorten protocols, reduce consumables, and enable decentralized imaging offers multiple pathways to lower the environmental impact of radiology. Yet these benefits are not automatic; they depend on deliberate design choices, targeted operational policies, and a willingness to integrate sustainability into performance metrics.

Achieving truly “green AI” in medical imaging requires more than efficient algorithms. It calls for a coordinated approach that spans model design, hardware selection, data management, infrastructure, and life cycle planning. Only by aligning these elements can AI become a powerful enabler of low-carbon, high-quality healthcare imaging.

## 8.4 Regulatory, Ethical, and Governance Perspectives

For AI in medical imaging to serve both patient care and planetary health, environmental sustainability must become a core consideration in its regulation, ethical framing, and governance. At present, sustainability remains largely peripheral to AI ethics, which has focused on fairness, transparency, privacy, and safety [74]. Given the resource demands of AI, from hardware manufacturing to model training and deployment, this omission is increasingly untenable.

### 8.4.1 Expanding Ethical Principles to Include Planetary Health

Traditional bioethical principles offer a clear pathway for embedding sustainability into AI governance. Transparency should extend beyond algorithmic decision-making to include full disclosure of the energy and water consumed in AI development and operation, the sourcing of materials for hardware, and the total carbon footprint across the AI life cycle.

Beneficence—the obligation to “do good”—must consider not only direct patient benefits but also wider public health implications. A diagnostic AI tool that benefits a narrow patient group while imposing a disproportionate carbon burden may not represent a net positive when viewed at the population level. Likewise, justice must go beyond equitable dataset representation to address the uneven global distribution of environmental harms. Mining rare earth elements for AI hardware often occurs in low-income countries, leaving local communities to bear ecological degradation and health risks, while the technology's benefits accrue primarily elsewhere [75].

Non-maleficence—avoiding harm—applies to environmental damage as well. AI systems that demand large-scale resource extraction, high electricity consumption, or water-intensive cooling indirectly contribute to climate change, air pollution, and water scarcity, all of which have measurable health consequences. Ignoring these harms risks perpetuating what has been described as "climate-related structural violence" [76].

### 8.4.2 Strengthening Standards, Reporting, and Accountability

Some progress has been made toward embedding sustainability into policy. The EU AI Act, which came into force in August 2024, acknowledges AI's role in environmental protection, though its provisions remain aspirational and lack enforceable performance thresholds [77]. The medical imaging industry has introduced EPDs for hardware and refurbishment standards that extend equipment lifespan (see Sect. 8.3.5), but equivalent tools for AI software are still missing. A radiology-specific eco-label, similar to "Energy Star" ratings, could enable hospitals to compare tools by both clinical and environmental performance.

Robust environmental reporting is essential for accountability. Journals, conferences, and funding bodies could require that developers disclose the environmental footprint of their AI models, including hardware specifications, compute hours, data center location, energy mix, and estimated $CO_2e$ emissions. Tools such as the *Machine Learning Emissions Calculator* [78] or *Carbontracker* [79] can facilitate this. Publishing such figures alongside accuracy metrics would make trade-offs transparent and encourage efficiency-focused innovation.

### 8.4.3 Broadening the Governance Lens

Sustainable AI governance requires expanding the scope of who is considered a stakeholder. Beyond clinicians, researchers, and developers, communities affected by resource extraction, e-waste processing, or the siting of large data centers should have a voice in decision-making. Including environmental scientists, sustainability experts, and public health professionals in advisory and regulatory bodies ensures that biodiversity, ecosystem integrity, and long-term climate impacts are considered alongside patient outcomes.

Multi-stakeholder platforms such as the Green AI Consortium and the Sustainable Healthcare Coalition [75] already demonstrate the value of collaborative approaches to setting standards and aligning innovation with environmental responsibility. Strengthening and expanding such initiatives could help harmonize sustainability practices across regions and health systems [75, 80].

**In short**, moving from voluntary commitments to enforceable obligations and broadening the ethical scope to explicitly include planetary health will ensure that AI in medical imaging delivers benefits not only for patients today but also for the environment and future generations.

## 8.5 Considerations Toward a Sustainable AI Future in Medical Imaging

The shift toward environmentally sustainable AI in medical imaging will require coordinated action across research, clinical practice, industry, and policy. It is not enough to rely on technical innovation alone; lasting change will come from integrating sustainability into the entire life cycle of AI tools (see Sect. 8.3), supported by governance (see Sect. 8.4), collaboration, and clear performance targets.

### 8.5.1 Designing and Deploying AI with Sustainability in Mind

Sustainability must be embedded from the earliest stages of AI design. This means selecting and optimizing model architectures not only for accuracy and robustness but also for computational efficiency, avoiding unnecessary complexity when leaner solutions achieve equivalent clinical outcomes. LCA should be a standard part of development pipelines, quantifying the environmental impact of proposed algorithms and workflows before deployment.

Technical strategies such as pruning, quantization, knowledge distillation, and transfer learning can significantly reduce the computational burden of training and inference. When coupled with energy-efficient hardware, such as TPUs, FPGAs, or low-power edge devices, these approaches minimize operational demands. AI can also directly support sustainability in clinical workflows, for example, by enabling shorter acquisition times, lower radiation doses, and reduced contrast agent use, all of which cut energy consumption and resource requirements.

Importantly, sustainability should extend into deployment decisions. AI-driven decision support can guide modality selection toward the lowest-carbon option that still meets diagnostic requirements, such as recommending ultrasound, low-dose CT, or abbreviated MRI examinations where appropriate. Providing clinicians with information about the estimated carbon footprint of alternative imaging strategies would further encourage environmentally conscious choices.

### 8.5.2 Embedding Transparency, Accountability, and Collaboration

Transparency in environmental performance is critical for accountability. Standardized metrics, such as energy consumption per scan, $CO_2e$ emissions per inference, and the life cycle impact of hardware, should be routinely measured, reported, and considered in procurement decisions. Funding agencies, journals, and regulators can accelerate adoption by making environmental reporting a requirement for AI research and deployment. Benchmarking datasets that incorporate both clinical and environmental performance would allow hospitals and researchers to compare solutions on multiple axes.

Progress will also depend on multi-stakeholder collaboration. Clinicians, AI developers, administrators, industry, policymakers, environmental scientists, and patient representatives all have a role in defining sustainability targets, sharing best practices, and coordinating investments. International platforms such as the Green AI Consortium and the Sustainable Healthcare Coalition already provide models for cross-sector cooperation, and expanding such initiatives could help align standards globally.

### 8.5.3 Driving Change Through Policy and Continuous Improvement

Voluntary measures alone are unlikely to achieve the speed or scale of change needed. Regulatory frameworks should include enforceable environmental performance standards for AI in medical imaging, alongside clear compliance pathways. Procurement policies can be a powerful lever, favoring products and services that meet verified sustainability criteria. Incentives such as preferential reimbursement for low-impact imaging workflows or carbon credits for meeting emissions targets could further accelerate uptake.

Finally, sustainability must be treated as an ongoing commitment rather than a one-off achievement. Continuous monitoring of AI systems and imaging workflows will ensure that environmental gains are maintained as technology, clinical practice, and climate challenges evolve. Education and training programs for radiologists, technologists, and AI engineers will be essential in fostering this culture, equipping future professionals to balance clinical and environmental priorities.

In essence, the path to sustainable AI in medical imaging rests on three pillars: designing with environmental efficiency as a core requirement, embedding transparency and collaboration into governance, and driving adoption through policy and ongoing optimization. By aligning these elements, the imaging community can ensure that AI delivers not only better diagnostics but also tangible benefits for planetary health.

## 8.6 Conclusion

AI in medical imaging is rapidly moving from experimental deployments to routine clinical use, offering unprecedented opportunities to improve diagnostic accuracy, accelerate workflows, and expand access to advanced imaging. Yet, these benefits come with a substantial environmental cost that spans the entire life cycle, from the extraction of raw materials for high-performance hardware, to the energy-intensive processes of model training and inference, to the eventual disposal or recycling of outdated equipment.

This chapter has shown that the environmental footprint of AI is not a fixed cost but a variable one, shaped by design choices, deployment strategies, and governance frameworks. Technical measures such as model compression, energy-efficient hardware, and AI-enabled scan acceleration can significantly reduce resource use, but only if sustainability is treated as a core performance criterion rather than an optional add-on. Similarly, policies that mandate environmental reporting, set measurable performance thresholds, and incentivize low-impact workflows can accelerate the shift toward greener practices.

The challenge now is to act collectively. Researchers must design algorithms that balance accuracy with efficiency; clinicians must incorporate sustainability into imaging decisions; industry must provide transparent environmental data for both hardware and software; and policymakers must create the regulatory conditions that make sustainable choices the default. The environmental crisis is both a health crisis and a technological one, and in medical imaging, AI is uniquely positioned to address both, if guided by the right principles.

By embedding environmental stewardship into the DNA of AI innovation, the imaging community can ensure that these technologies not only enhance patient care today but also help safeguard the health of the planet for future generations. Sustainable AI in medical imaging is not a distant aspiration; it is a necessity, and the path forward is already within our reach.

## References


1. Wolf RM, Abramoff MD, Channa R, Tava C, Clarida W, Lehmann HP. Potential reduction in healthcare carbon footprint by autonomous artificial intelligence. NPJ Digit Med. 2022;5(1):62.
2. Cho R. AI's growing carbon footprint. Volume 20252023.
3. Monserrate SG. The staggering ecological impacts of computation and the cloud. Volume 20252022.
4. Yañez-Barnuevo M. Data centers and water consumption. Volume 20252025.
5. Picano E, Mangia C, D'Andrea A. Climate change, carbon dioxide emissions, and medical imaging contribution. J Clin Med. 2022;12(1)
6. Afat S, Wohlers J, Herrmann J, Brendlin AS, Gassenmaier S, Almansour H, Werner S, Brendel JM, Mika A, Scherieble C, Notohamiprodjo M, Gatidis S, Nikolaou K, Küstner T. Reducing energy consumption in musculoskeletal MRI using shorter scan protocols, optimized magnet cooling patterns, and deep learning sequences. Eur Radiol. 2025;35(4):1993–2004.
7. Heye T, Knoerl R, Wehrle T, Mangold D, Cerminara A, Loser M, Plumeyer M, Degen M, Lüthy R, Brodbeck D, Merkle E. The energy consumption of radiology: energy- and cost-saving opportunities for CT and MRI operation. Radiology. 2020;295(3):593–605.
8. Brünjes R, Hofmann T. Anthropogenic gadolinium in freshwater and drinking water systems. Water Res. 2020;182:115966.
9. Doo FX, Vosshenrich J, Cook TS, Moy L, Almeida E, Woolen SA, Gichoya JW, Heye T, Hanneman K. Environmental sustainability and AI in radiology: a double-edged sword. Radiology. 2024;310(2):e232030.
10. Pennar K. 'If I were a hospital, I'd be reading the tea leaves': pressures grow on the health care industry to reduce its climate pollution. Volume 20252022.
11. Wagner F, Raab F, Varadarajan S, Gühring J, Schneider R, Herrmann J, Nikolaou K, Afat S, Küstner T. Optimizing energy efficiency in MRI scanners: a workflow analysis for enhanced sustainability. 2025.
12. Raab F, Wagner F, Wohlers J, Varadarajan S, Gühring J, Schneider R, Herrmann J, Notohamiprodjo M, Nikolaou K, Afat S. Optimizing energy efficiency in MRI scanners. MAGNETOM Flash. 2025;91(2):17–22.
13. Chaban YV, Vosshenrich J, McKee H, Gunasekaran S, Brown MJ, Atalay MK, Heye T, Markl M, Woolen SA, Simonetti OP, Hanneman

K. Environmental sustainability and MRI: challenges, opportunities, and a call for action. J Magn Reson Imaging. 2024;59(4):1149–67.
14. Barloese M, Petersen CL. Sustainable health care: a real-world appraisal of a modern imaging department. Clin Imaging. 2024;105:110025.
15. Hanneman K, McKee H, Nguyen ET, Panet H, Kielar A. Greenhouse gas emissions by diagnostic imaging modality in a hospital-based radiology department. Can Assoc Radiol J. 2024;75(4):950–3.
16. McAlister S, McGain F, Petersen M, Story D, Charlesworth K, Ison G, Barratt A. The carbon footprint of hospital diagnostic imaging in Australia. Lancet Reg Health West Pac. 2022;24:100459.
17. Cowls J, Tsamados A, Taddeo M, Floridi L. The AI gambit: leveraging artificial intelligence to combat climate change-opportunities, challenges, and recommendations. AI Soc. 2023;38(1):283–307.
18. Jiang P, Sonne C, Li W, You F, You S. Preventing the immense increase in the life-cycle energy and carbon footprints of LLM-powered intelligent Chatbots. Engineering. 2024;40:202–10.
19. Kjelle E, Andersen ER, Krokeide AM, Soril LJJ, van Bodegom-Vos L, Clement FM, Hofmann BM. Characterizing and quantifying low-value diagnostic imaging internationally: a scoping review. BMC Med Imaging. 2022;22(1):73.
20. Kjelle E, Andersen ER, Soril LJJ, van Bodegom-Vos L, Hofmann BM. Interventions to reduce low-value imaging—a systematic review of interventions and outcomes. BMC Health Serv Res. 2021;21(1):983.
21. Kjelle E, Brandsæter I, Andersen ER, Hofmann BM. Cost of low-value imaging worldwide: a systematic review. Appl Health Econ Health Policy. 2024;22(4):485–501.
22. Hofmann B. Low-value imaging: concept analysis and definition. Eur J Radiol. 2025;183:111858.
23. Brandsæter IØ, Andersen ER, Hofmann BM, Kjelle E. Drivers for low-value imaging: a qualitative study of stakeholders' perspectives in Norway. BMC Health Serv Res. 2023;23(1):295.
24. Andersen ER, Brandsæter IØ, Hofmann BM, Kjelle E. The use of low-value imaging: the role of referral practice and access to imaging services in a representative area of Norway. Insights Imaging. 2023;14(1):29.
25. Kjelle E, Brandsæter IØ, Andersen ER, Hofmann B. Sustainability in healthcare by reducing low-value imaging – a narrative review. Radiography. 2024;30:30–4.
26. Prince EW, Mirsky DM, Hankinson TC, Görg C. Impact of AI decision support on clinical experts' radiographic interpretation of Adamantinomatous Craniopharyngioma. AMIA Annu Symp Proc. 2024;2024:930–9.
27. Yan TD, Jalal S, Harris A. Value-based radiology in Canada: reducing low-value care and improving system efficiency. Can Assoc Radiol J. 2025;76(1):61–7.

28. Woolen SA, Deshpande V, Becker AE, Dai S, Su P, Itriago-Leon P, Huang SY, Tabari A, Hanneman K, Vosshenrich J, Hess CP, Martin AJ. Low-carbon MRI: acceleration strategies to reduce emissions and expand imaging capacity. Radiology. 2025;315(1):e243453.
29. Hammernik K, Küstner T, Yaman B, Huang Z, Rueckert D, Knoll F, Akçakaya M. Physics-driven deep learning for computational magnetic resonance imaging: combining physics and machine learning for improved medical imaging. IEEE Signal Process Mag. 2023;40(1):98–114.
30. Heckel R, Jacob M, Chaudhari A, Perlman O, Shimron E. Deep learning for accelerated and robust MRI reconstruction. MAGMA. 2024;37(3):335–68.
31. Glessgen C, Crowe LA, Wetzl J, Schmidt M, Yoon SS, Vallée JP, Deux JF. Automated vs manual cardiac MRI planning: a single-center prospective evaluation of reliability and scan times. Eur Radiol. 2025;35(7):3927–36.
32. Silva SN, Woodgate T, McElroy S, Cleri M, Clair KS, Verdera JA, Payette K, Uus A, Story L, Lloyd D, Rutherford MA, Hajnal JV, Pushparajah K, Hutter J. Automatic flow planning for fetal cardiovascular magnetic resonance imaging. J Cardiovasc Magn Reson. 2025;27(1):101888.
33. Emami H, Dong M, Nejad-Davarani SP, Glide-Hurst CK. SA-GAN: structure-aware GAN for organ-preserving synthetic CT generation. Springer; 2021. p. 471–81.
34. Pan S, Abouei E, Wynne J, Chang CW, Wang T, Qiu RL, Li Y, Peng J, Roper J, Patel P. Synthetic CT generation from MRI using 3D transformer-based denoising diffusion model. Med Phys. 2024;51(4):2538–48.
35. Kofler A, Si D, Schote D, Botnar RM, Kolbitsch C, Prieto C. MR imaging in the low-field: Leveraging the power of machine learning. 2025. arXiv preprint arXiv:250117211.
36. Koonjoo N, Zhu B, Bagnall GC, Bhutto D, Rosen MS. Boosting the signal-to-noise of low-field MRI with deep learning image reconstruction. Sci Rep. 2021;11(1):8248.
37. Ayde R, Vornehm M, Zhao Y, Knoll F, Wu EX, Sarracanie M. MRI at low field: a review of software solutions for improving SNR. NMR Biomed. 2025;38(1):e5268.
38. Haubold J, Hosch R, Umutlu L, Wetter A, Haubold P, Radbruch A, Forsting M, Nensa F, Koitka S. Contrast agent dose reduction in computed tomography with deep learning using a conditional generative adversarial network. Eur Radiol. 2021;31(8):6087–95.
39. Yonathan G, Afom Tesfalem A, Melino N, Chase Y. Bridging the AI gap in clinical imaging: opportunities and strategies for low- and middle-income countries. J Glob Radiol. 2025;11(2)
40. Achour N, Zapata T, Saleh Y, Pierscionek B, Azzopardi-Muscat N, Novillo-Ortiz D, Morgan C, Chaouali M. The role of AI in mitigating the

impact of radiologist shortages: a systematised review. Health Technol (Berl). 2025;15(3):489–501.

41. East SA, Wang Y, Yanamala N, Maganti K, Sengupta PP. Artificial intelligence-enabled point-of-care echocardiography: bringing precision imaging to the bedside. Curr Atheroscler Rep. 2025;27(1):70.
42. Kim S, Fischetti C, Guy M, Hsu E, Fox J, Young SD. Artificial intelligence (AI) applications for Point of Care Ultrasound (POCUS) in low-resource settings: a scoping review. Diagnostics (Basel). 2024;14(15)
43. Martin M, Mohnke A, Lewis GM, Dunnick NR, Keoleian G, Maturen KE. Environmental impacts of abdominal imaging: a pilot investigation. J Am Coll Radiol. 2018;15(10):1385–93.
44. Picano E, Mangia C, D'Andrea A. Climate change, carbon dioxide emissions, and medical imaging contribution. J Clin Med. 2023;12(1):215.
45. McAlister S, Barratt A, Bell K, McGain F. How many carbon emissions are saved by doing one less MRI? Lancet Planet Heath. 2024;8(6):e350.
46. Shokoohi H, Liteplo AS, Montoya K, Patnode C, Hutchinson AB, Zalis ME, Gottlieb M, Raja AS, Slutzman JE. Climate-smart diagnostic medical imaging and point-of-care ultrasound: an evidence-based perspective. J Emerg Med. 2025;75:150–7.
47. Anudjo MNK, Vitale C, Elshami W, Hancock A, Adeleke S, Franklin JM, Akudjedu TN. Considerations for environmental sustainability in clinical radiology and radiotherapy practice: a systematic literature review and recommendations for a greener practice. Radiography. 2023;29(6):1077–92.
48. Rockall AG, Allen B, Brown MJ, El-Diasty T, Fletcher J, Gerson RF, Goergen S, Marrero González AP, Grist TM, Hanneman K, Hess CP, Ho ELM, Salama DH, Schoen J, Sheard S. Sustainability in radiology: position paper and call to action from ACR, AOSR, ASR, CAR, CIR, ESR, ESRNM, ISR, IS3R, RANZCR, and RSNA. Radiology. 2025;314(3):e250325.
49. Li J, Mao Y, Zhang J. Maintenance and quality control of medical equipment based on information fusion technology. Comput Intell Neurosci. 2022;2022(1):9333328.
50. Lekadir K, Osuala R, Gallin C, Lazrak N, Kushibar K, Tsakou G, Aussó S, Alberich LC, Marias K, Tsiknakis M. FUTURE-AI: guiding principles and consensus recommendations for trustworthy artificial intelligence in medical imaging. 2021. arXiv preprint arXiv:210909658.
51. Global Electronics C. State of sustainability research for medical imaging equipment. Portland: Global Electronics Council; 2022.
52. Roletto A, Zanardo M, Bonfitto GR, Catania D, Sardanelli F, Zanoni S. The environmental impact of energy consumption and carbon emissions in radiology departments: a systematic review. Eur Radiol Exp. 2024;8(1):35.

53. Han S, Mao H, Dally WJ. Deep compression: compressing deep neural networks with pruning, trained quantization and huffman coding. 2015. arXiv preprint arXiv:151000149.
54. Jacob B, Kligys S, Chen B, Zhu M, Tang M, Howard A, Adam H, Kalenichenko D. Quantization and training of neural networks for efficient integer-arithmetic-only inference. 2018. pp. 2704–2713.
55. Hinton G, Vinyals O, Dean J. Distilling the knowledge in a neural network. 2015. arXiv preprint arXiv:150302531.
56. Pan SJ, Yang Q. A survey on transfer learning. IEEE Trans Knowl Data Eng. 2009;22(10):1345–59.
57. Yang T-J, Chen Y-H, Sze V. Designing energy-efficient convolutional neural networks using energy-aware pruning. 2017. pp. 5687–5695.
58. Caldeira E, Neto PC, Huber M, Damer N, Sequeira AF. Model compression techniques in biometrics applications: a survey. Inf Fusion. 2025;114:102657.
59. Violos J, Diamanti K-C, Kompatsiaris I, Papadopoulos S. Frugal machine learning for energy-efficient, and resource-aware Artificial Intelligence. 2025. arXiv preprint arXiv:250601869.
60. Rafat K, Islam S, Mahfug AA, Hossain MI, Rahman F, Momen S, Rahman S, Mohammed N. Mitigating carbon footprint for knowledge distillation based deep learning model compression. PLoS One. 2023;18(5):e0285668.
61. Corral JMR, Civit-Masot J, Luna-Perejón F, Díaz-Cano I, Morgado-Estévez A, Domínguez-Morales M. Energy efficiency in edge TPU vs. embedded GPU for computer-aided medical imaging segmentation and classification. Eng Appl Artif Intell. 2024;127:107298.
62. Marković D, Grollier J. Quantum neuromorphic computing. Appl Phys Lett. 2020;117:15.
63. Harvey C, Clark S, Brown D, Meichanetzidis K. Learning complex word embeddings in classical and quantum spaces. 2024. arXiv preprint arXiv:241213745.
64. Xu W, Clark S, Brown D, Matos G, Meichanetzidis K. Quantum recurrent architectures for text classification, pp. 18020–18027. 2024.
65. Khatri N, Matos G, Coopmans L, Clark S. Quixer: a quantum transformer model. 2024. arXiv preprint arXiv:240604305.
66. Harvey C, Yeung R, Meichanetzidis K. Sequence processing with quantum tensor networks. 2023. arXiv preprint arXiv:230807865.
67. Heydari S, Mahmoud QH. Tiny machine learning and on-device inference: a survey of applications, challenges, and future directions. Sensors. 2025;25(10):3191.
68. Konečný J, McMahan HB, Ramage D, Richtárik P. Federated optimization: distributed machine learning for on-device intelligence. 2016. arXiv preprint arXiv:161002527.

69. Amazon. AWS for Healthcare at ECR 2025: Advancing Sustainable Medical Imaging. 2025. p https://aws.amazon.com/de/blogs/industries/aws-for-healthcare-at-ecr-2025-advancing-sustainable-medical-imaging/
70. Kocak B, Ponsiglione A, Romeo V, Ugga L, Huisman M, Cuocolo R. Radiology AI and sustainability paradox: environmental, economic, and social dimensions. Insights Imaging. 2025;16(1):88.
71. Zhang X, Lindberg T, Xiong N, Vyatkin V, Mousavi A. Cooling energy consumption investigation of data center IT room with vertical placed server. Energy Procedia. 2017;105:2047–52.
72. Thangam D, Muniraju H, Ramesh R, Narasimhaiah R, Muddasir Ahamed Khan N, Booshan S, Booshan B, Manickam T, Sankar GR. Impact of data centers on power consumption, climate change, and sustainability. In: Kumar KD, Varadarajan V, Nasser N, Poluru RK, editors. Computational intelligence for green cloud computing and digital waste management. Hershey: IGI Global Scientific Publishing; 2024. p. 60–83.
73. Masanet E, Lei N. How much energy do data centers really use? Volume 20252020.
74. Luccioni AS, Pistilli G, Sefala R, Moorosi N. Bridging the gap: integrating ethics and environmental sustainability in AI research and practice. 2025. arXiv preprint arXiv:250400797.
75. Ueda D, Walston SL, Fujita S, Fushimi Y, Tsuboyama T, Kamagata K, Yamada A, Yanagawa M, Ito R, Fujima N, Kawamura M, Nakaura T, Matsui Y, Tatsugami F, Fujioka T, Nozaki T, Hirata K, Naganawa S. Climate change and artificial intelligence in healthcare: review and recommendations towards a sustainable future. Diagn Interv Imaging. 2024;105(11):453–9.
76. Fiske A, Radhuber IM, Willem T, Buyx A, Celi LA, McLennan S. Climate change and health: the next challenge of ethical AI. Lancet Glob Health. 2025;13(7):e1314–20.
77. Union E. Artificial Intelligence Act (AI Act). Volume 20252024.
78. Lacoste A, Luccioni A, Schmidt V, Dandres T. Quantifying the carbon emissions of machine learning. 2019. arXiv preprint arXiv:191009700.
79. Anthony LFW, Kanding B, Selvan R. Carbontracker: tracking and predicting the carbon footprint of training deep learning models. 2020. arXiv preprint arXiv:200703051.
80. Bachina L, Kanagala A, Korapu S, Ratnaraju P. Sustainable materials for artificial intelligence (AI) technology adoption for energy-efficient patient-centric healthcare solutions. J Educ Health Promot. 2025;14:4.

# List of Case Studies and Examples

The examples are categorized into the environmental challenges driving the need for sustainable AI (footprint) and the specific AI/operational solutions being implemented or proposed (interventions).

## Environmental Footprint and Resource Consumption (The Challenge)

These examples quantify the environmental challenge that the book seeks to address:

| Category | Case study/example | Supporting sources |
|---|---|---|
| Global emissions & radiology contribution | CT and MR imaging were estimated to contribute up to **0.77% of total global carbon dioxide emissions** in 2016 [1]. Medical imaging is broadly estimated to account for about **1% of total global $CO_2$ emissions** [2, 3] | [1–3] |
| Radiology energy use (MRI/CT) | Annual energy consumption for a modern MRI unit ranges from **80,000 to 170,000 kWh** [4, 5]. A single MRI scanner consumes, on average, more than **100 MWh annually**, making it the most energy-intensive device in radiology [4, 5]. CT scanners consume **20,000–35,000 kWh** annually [5] | [4, 5] |

(continued)


E. R. Ranschaert et al. (eds.), *Sustainability of AI in Radiology*, Imaging Informatics for Healthcare Professionals,
https://doi.org/10.1007/978-3-032-15693-8

| Category | Case study/example | Supporting sources |
|---|---|---|
| Idle equipment waste | Radiology departments waste **40–91% of energy usage** in nonproductive states [6, 7]. For CT, the majority of energy consumption (**around two-thirds**) occurs during the system's nonproductive idle state [7]. Even in "system-off" mode, MRI units consume **31–38% of their annual energy** to maintain magnet superconductivity [5, 8] | [5–8] |
| Manufacturing footprint | Manufacturing a single **MRI machine** consumes about **753,000 kWh** of fossil fuel energy [9] or **792,100 kg $CO_2$ equivalent** [9] | [9] |
| Material waste | Interventional radiology procedures produce an average of **8 kg of waste per case** [10]. More than **ten million liters** of iodinated contrast media (ICM) are used globally every year [11] | [10, 11] |
| Contrast agent contamination | An estimated **19 tons of gadolinium** enter EU wastewater annually [12]. The presence of ICM and gadolinium-based contrast agents (GBCA) has been confirmed in **surface water, groundwater, and drinking water** worldwide [11–13] | [11–13] |
| AI training costs (energy and carbon) | Training **GPT-3** required **1287 MWh** and is estimated to have emitted **552 tons of $CO_2$** [14, 15]. Training large models can produce emissions equivalent to the lifetime emissions of **several gasoline-powered cars** [3] | [3, 14, 15] |
| Water footprint | Training **GPT-3** may have used **700,000 L** of freshwater, primarily for cooling the servers [16]. Globally, data centers consume around **626 billion gallons** of water per year [17] | [16, 17] |

## AI and Operational Interventions (The Solution)

These examples highlight practical and proposed actions for enhancing sustainability in clinical, technological, and regulatory domains:

| Category | Case study/example | Supporting sources |
|---|---|---|
| AI-enabled scan reduction | **AI-based image reconstruction** reduces scan times by **30–50%** [3]. AI-accelerated sequences have been shown to reduce scan times by up to **71%** and energy use by **72%** in musculoskeletal MRI [8]. Accelerating protocols by 25–75% across a practice was projected to save **200.6–867.1 MWh** annually [8] | [3, 8] |
| AI for efficiency (utilization) | Switching MRI scanners from idle to off overnight reduced energy use by **25–33%** annually [18]. Increasing scanner utilization from 30% to 90% yielded a nearly **threefold reduction** in per-patient energy consumption [19] | [18, 19] |
| AI synthesis (contrast reduction) | The **NetZeroAICT project** is an EU-funded initiative developing AI-driven technology to synthesize contrast-enhanced images from non-contrast CTs [20]. AI can cut iodinated contrast usage in CT by up to **50%** [21] or enable **virtual native enhancement** in MRI [3] | [3, 20, 21] |
| AI synthesis (modality conversion) | Deep learning models have shown the feasibility of generating **synthetic CT from MRI** for radiotherapy planning [22, 23] | [22, 23] |
| Contrast agent alternatives | **Ultra-small superparamagnetic iron oxide particles (USPIOs)** are an alternative to GBCA [24]. Follow-up of conditions like **vestibular schwannomas and meningiomas** can be performed without contrast media [25, 26] | [24–26] |

(continued)

| Category | Case study/example | Supporting sources |
|---|---|---|
| Contrast agent collection | **Pilot studies in the Netherlands and Germany** have used disposable urine bags for outpatients to collect contrast media [27, 28]. The **Greenwater study** in Italy recovered **51.2% of ICM and 12.9% of GBCA** by asking outpatients to stay longer [29] | [27–29] |
| AI model efficiency (optimization) | A case study on **axSpA classification** found optimized 2D ResNet models consumed **0.31–0.33 kWh** for training, compared to energy-intensive 3D models which exceeded **1.58 kWh** [30] | [30] |
| Green computing infrastructure | **Google Cloud** has matched all its annual electricity use with an equivalent amount of **renewable energy since 2017** [31] | [31] |
| Governance/ standards | The **European Society of Radiology (ESR) GreenID Certification** is a structured sustainability accreditation scheme, piloted in **22 hospitals** [32, 33]. The **MeGadoRe Project** (France) focuses on **recycling gadolinium** [34] | [32–34] |
| Regulatory innovation | The **FDA'S Predetermined Change Control Plan (PCCP)** allows manufacturers to define preapproved updates for adaptive AI systems without repeated, time-consuming re-certification [35, 36] | [35, 36] |

# Glossary

**AI Act (EU)** The European Union Regulation on Artificial Intelligence, a legislative framework that categorizes AI systems by risk level and sets strict requirements for high-risk systems (including healthcare AI) concerning security, transparency, traceability, and human oversight.

**Anthropocene** The current geological age, in which the changes in the planet's environment are increasingly attributed to humanity's actions.

**Artificial intelligence (AI)** A growing influence in daily life, often involving algorithms that learn directly from data (machine learning) to perform tasks like detection, classification, and optimization in healthcare and radiology.

**Artificial neural networks (ANNs)** The basis of modern AI and deep learning; algorithms loosely inspired by the human brain that use sequentially connected layers of neurons containing trainable weights to perform mathematical operations.

**Carbon footprint ($CO_2$e)** A key sustainability metric used to measure the total carbon dioxide equivalent emissions generated throughout the life cycle of AI systems, radiological equipment, or the entire healthcare sector.

**Carbontracker** A tool/software package used to provide real-time tracking of energy consumption during AI training cycles, enabling researchers to estimate emissions.


E. R. Ranschaert et al. (eds.), *Sustainability of AI in Radiology*, Imaging Informatics for Healthcare Professionals,
https://doi.org/10.1007/978-3-032-15693-8

**Clinical decision support (CDS)** Systems, often AI-enabled, that provide real-time guidance to clinicians at the point of care to help inform decisions about a patient's care, potentially reducing inappropriate imaging orders.

**Cloud computing** Data storage and processing solutions where services are provided over the Internet. Can offer scalability but involves energy costs related to continuous data transmission and remote processing.

**Convolutional neural networks (CNNs)** An advanced architecture of ANNs commonly used in image analysis. They exploit relationships between neighboring pixels by using convolutional layers to calculate features like edges and lines.

**Contrast media (CM)** Agents used in CT (iodinated contrast media, ICM) and MRI (gadolinium-based contrast agents, GBCA) to enhance image detail. Their extensive use contributes significantly to water contamination and environmental burden.

**Data life cycle management** Policies ensuring that obsolete or redundant datasets are identified and deleted, reducing the energy required to maintain unused data and minimizing the environmental toll of digital infrastructure.

**Dark data** Data that is collected but never used, consuming energy without delivering operational or analytical value; estimates suggest over half of an organization's stored data falls into this category.

**Deep learning (DL)** A subset of machine learning algorithms that use artificial neural networks with multiple layers (a "deep" structure).

**Diffusion models** A current state-of-the-art method in generative AI for photorealistic image generation, trained to perform the inverse operation of gradually adding noise to an image.

**Electronic waste (e-waste)** Waste generated from discarded electronic equipment (e.g., computers, GPUs, imaging systems) which requires substantial energy to manufacture and can contain hazardous materials.

**Energy star** A US Environmental Protection Agency product specification developed for medical imaging equipment to allow for transparency and informed sustainable purchasing decisions.

**Environmental, Social, Governance (ESG)** A framework that is increasingly reflected in regulatory expectations, encompassing environmental impacts, social justice, equitable access to care, and transparency of technological decision-making.

**European Health Data Space (EHDS)** An EU initiative working to create a harmonized environment for sharing health data between Member States, supporting the secure development of AI systems while adhering to GDPR principles.

**Federated learning** An approach that allows the training of AI models across multiple decentralized devices or institutions without the need to centralize sensitive health data, enhancing data privacy and reducing transfer emissions.

**Foundation models** Large-scale AI models trained on massive amounts of data, usually in a self-supervised way, designed to adapt to many down-stream tasks. They are typically larger and more energy-intensive than task-specific models.

**Gadolinium-based contrast agents (GBCA)** MRI contrast media whose excretion into sewage water raises environmental concerns due to their presence in aquatic environments.

**Generative AI** The area of AI focused on generating new data samples (e.g., images or text) based on patterns learned during training, utilizing methods like diffusion models and GANs.

**Generative adversarial network (GAN)** A generative AI method consisting of a generator and a discriminator network that compete against each other to produce realistic samples.

**Green AI** A concept treating efficiency and reduced environmental footprint as fundamental aspects of AI evaluation, balancing clinical gains against resource consumption.

**Green team** An imaging sustainability group or committee established within a department, consisting of diverse staff roles (radiologists, radiographers, policy officers, etc.) to drive and integrate sustainable practices effectively.

**Iodinated contrast media (ICM)** Contrast media most frequently used in CT scans; millions of liters are used globally every year, contributing to environmental contamination.

**Inference** The actual use or running of a trained AI model (making predictions), which has a much lower individual energy expenditure than training, but cumulative inference costs can quickly surpass training emissions due to frequent use.

**Knowledge distillation** An algorithmic strategy where knowledge is transferred from a large, complex "teacher" model into a smaller, simpler "student" model, resulting in smaller models that require less computational power and energy for deployment.

**Life cycle analysis (LCA)** A methodology that quantifies environmental impacts from raw material extraction through manufacturing, operation, and end-of-life disposal of devices or AI systems, essential for understanding the full environmental cost.

**Low-value imaging** Imaging tests that provide little or no clinical benefit while consuming energy and resources. AI-enabled Clinical Decision Support (CDS) aims to reduce this activity.

**MDR/IVDR** European regulations (Medical Device Regulation/ In Vitro Diagnostic Regulation) that define minimum requirements for documentation management, audit trails, and change management of medical devices, including AI systems.

**Net zero emissions** The goal of achieving a balance between the amount of greenhouse gas emitted and the amount removed from the atmosphere, often cited as the target for sustainable healthcare and AI.

**Neuromorphic computing** Emerging technologies that promise greater reductions in energy demand than conventional hardware, offering a path toward sustainable AI.

**Overfitting** A risk during the AI training process where a network performs much better on the training data than on new, unseen data.

**Picture Archiving and Communication Systems (PACS)** Systems used in radiology departments for image processing, storage, and interpretation, running on high-performance PCs that contribute to energy demands.

**Predetermined Change Control Plan (PCCP)** A regulatory concept supported by the FDA for adaptive AI systems that can dynamically change after launch. It allows manufacturers to define preapproved updates without requiring re-certification, reducing regulatory burden.

**Pruning** An algorithmic strategy to simplify AI models by removing unnecessary components (redundant weights or neurons), which reduces computational overhead and improves efficiency.

**Quantization** An algorithmic strategy that reduces the precision of numerical values (e.g., from 32-bit floating-point to 8-bit integers) in AI computations, significantly lowering memory and compute demand during inference.

**Radiomics** The use of AI to transform medical images into quantitative biomarkers, valuable for personalized medicine and prognosis.

**Renewable energy** Energy sources like wind and solar used to power data centers, which can dramatically reduce the carbon footprint associated with AI training and operation.

**Sustainability by design** The principle of taking long-term sustainability into account when designing AI systems, ensuring they meet not just minimum requirements but also actively consider environmental and social impacts across the entire life cycle.

**Training** The iterative process of adjusting the tunable parameters (weights) in a neural network using a dedicated training set with the objective of minimizing the loss function. This phase is typically the most energy-intensive part of AI development.

**Transparency** The ethical principle requiring open disclosure of an AI system's decision-making process, data use, and governance, expanded in the "third wave" of AI ethics to include the full disclosure of the system's environmental footprint.

**U-Net** A neural network architecture particularly well-suited for medical image segmentation, known for its use of skip connections, allowing it to achieve high accuracy with limited training data.

**Water footprint (usage)** A critical, often hidden, environmental cost of AI and data centers, referring to the large amounts of water required for cooling servers and generating electricity.

# Bibliography


1. Rockall AG, Allen B, Brown MJ, El-Diasty T, Fletcher J, Gerson RF, Goergen S, Marrero González AP, Grist TM, Hanneman K, Hess CP, Ho ELM, Salama DH, Schoen J, Sheard S. Sustainability in radiology: position paper and call to action from ACR, AOSR, ASR, CAR, CIR, ESR, ESRNM, ISR, IS3R, RANZCR and RSNA. Eur Radiol. 2025;35:5427–36.
2. Picano E, Mangia C, D'Andrea A. Climate change, carbon dioxide emissions, and medical imaging contribution. J Clin Med. 2022:12(1).
3. Doo FX, Vosshenrich J, Cook TS, Moy L, Almeida EPRP, Woolen SA, Gichoya JW, Heye T, Hanneman K. Environmental sustainability and AI in radiology: a double-edged sword. Radiology. 2024;310:e232030.
4. Afat S, Wohlers J, Herrmann J, Brendlin AS, Gassenmaier S, Almansour H, Werner S, Brendel JM, Mika A, Scherieble C, Notohamiprodjo M, Gatidis S, Nikolaou K, Küstner T. Reducing energy consumption in musculoskeletal MRI using shorter scan protocols, optimized magnet cooling patterns, and deep learning sequences. Eur Radiol. 2025;35(4):1993–2004.
5. Heye T, Knoerl R, Wehrle T, Mangold D, Cerminara A, Loser M, Plumeyer M, Degen M, Lüthy R, Brodbeck D, Merkle E. The energy consumption of radiology: energy- and cost-saving opportunities for CT and MRI operation. Radiology. 2020;295:192084.
6. Roletto A, Zanardo M, Bonfitto GR, Catania D, Sardanelli F, Zanoni S. The environmental impact of energy consumption and carbon emissions in radiology departments: a systematic review. Eur Radiol Exp. 2024;8:35.
7. Heye T, Knoerl R, Wehrle T, Mangold D, Cerminara A, Loser M, Plumeyer M, Degen M, Lüthy R, Brodbeck D, Merkle E. The energy consumption of radiology: energy- and cost-saving opportunities for CT and MRI operation. Radiology. 2020;295(3):593–605.



E. R. Ranschaert et al. (eds.), *Sustainability of AI in Radiology*, Imaging Informatics for Healthcare Professionals, https://doi.org/10.1007/978-3-032-15693-8

8. Woolen SA, Deshpande V, Becker AE, Dai S, Su P, Itriago-Leon P, Huang SY, Tabari A, Hanneman K, Vosshenrich J, Hess CP, Martin AJ. Low-carbon MRI: acceleration strategies to reduce emissions and expand imaging capacity. Radiology. 2025;315(1):e243453.
9. Martin M, Mohnke A, Lewis GM, Dunnick NR, Keoleian G, Maturen KE. Environmental impacts of abdominal imaging: a pilot investigation. J Am Coll Radiol. 2018;15(10):1385–93.
10. Woolen SA, Kim CJ, Hernandez AM, Becker A, Martin AJ, Kuoy E, Pevec WC, Tutton S. Radiology environmental impact: what is known and how can we improve? Acad Radiol. 2023;30:625–30.
11. Dekker HM, Stroomberg GJ, Prokop M. Tackling the increasing contamination of the water supply by iodinated contrast media. Insights Imaging. 2022;13:30.
12. Brünjes R, Hofmann T. Anthropogenic gadolinium in freshwater and drinking water systems. Water Res. 2020;182:115966.
13. Sengar A, Vijayanandan A. Comprehensive review on iodinated X-ray contrast media: complete fate, occurrence, and formation of disinfection byproducts. Sci Total Environ. 2021;769:144846.
14. Patterson D, Gonzalez J, Le Q, Liang C, Munguia LM, Rothchild D, et al. Carbon emissions and large neural network training. arXiv. 2021. Available from: http://arxiv.org/abs/2104.10350.
15. Thangam D, Muniraju H, Ramesh R, Narasimhaiah R, Muddasir N, Khan A, et al. Impact of data centers on power consumption, climate change, and sustainability. 2024.
16. Li P, Yang J, Islam MA, Ren S. Making AI less "thirsty": uncovering and addressing the secret water footprint of AI models. arXiv (2023): 2304.03271.
17. Yañez-Barnuevo M. Data centers and water consumption. Volume 20252025.
18. Woolen SA, Becker AE, Martin AJ, et al. Ecodesign and operational strategies to reduce the carbon footprint of MRI for energy cost savings. Radiology. 2023;307(4):e230441.
19. McKee H, Brown MJ, Kim HHR, Doo FX, Panet H, Rockall AG, et al. Planetary health and radiology: why we should care and what we can do. Radiology. 2024;311(1):e240219.
20. NetZeroAICT Consortium. NetZeroAICT: Digital Contrast for Computerised Tomography. Horizon Europe-funded research project (Grant No. 101136679); project webpage. 2025. Available from: https://netzeroaict.eu/
21. Haubold J, Hosch R, Umutlu L, Wetter A, Haubold P, Radbruch A, Forsting M, Nensa F, Koitka S. Contrast agent dose reduction in computed tomography with deep learning using a conditional generative adversarial network. Eur Radiol. 2021;31(8):6087–95.
22. Han X. MR-based synthetic CT generation using a deep convolutional neural network method. Med Phys. 2017;44(4):1408–19.

23. Pan S, Abouei E, Wynne J, Chang CW, Wang T, Qiu RL, Li Y, Peng J, Roper J, Patel P. Synthetic CT generation from MRI using 3D transformer—based denoising diffusion model. Med Phys. 2024;51(4):2538–48.
24. Dekker HM, Stroomberg GJ, Van der Molen AJ, Prokop M. Review of strategies to reduce the contamination of the water environment by gadolinium-based contrast agents. Insights Imaging. 2024;15(1):62.
25. Kim DH, Lee S, Hwang SH. Non-contrast magnetic resonance imaging for diagnosis and monitoring of vestibular Schwannomas: a systematic review and meta-analysis. Otol Neurotol. 2019;40(9):1126–33.
26. Rahatli FK, Donmez FY, Kesim C, Haberal KM, Turnaoglu H, Agildere AM. Can unenhanced brain magnetic resonance imaging be used in routine follow up of meningiomas to avoid gadolinium deposition in brain? Clin Imaging. 2019;53:155–61.
27. Hoogenboom J, Bergema K, van Vliet BJM, Hendriksen A. Eindrapportage Brede Plaszakkenproef. 2021.
28. Röntgenkrontrastmittel in der Ruhr: Pilotproject. www.merkmal-ruhr.de
29. Zanardo M, Ambrogi F, Asmundo L, Cardani R, Cirillo G, Colarieti A, Cozzi A, Cressoni M, Dambra I, Di Leo G, Monti CB, Nicotera L, Pomati F, Renna LV, Secchi F, Versuraro M, Vitali P, Sardanelli F. The GREEN-WATER study: patients' green sensitivity and potential recovery of injected contrast agents. Eur Radiol. 2025;35(3):1205–14.
30. Excerpt from Chapter 5 (Table 3: Model development experiments for axSPa classification).
31. Excerpt from Chapter 5 (Mention of Google Cloud matching its annual electricity use with an equivalent amount of renewable energy since 2017).
32. HealthManagement.org. Guiding radiology to a greener future. 2025. https://healthmanagement.org/c/imaging/News/guiding-radiology-to-a-greener-future.
33. Excerpt from Chapter 1 (ESR GreenID Certification pilot in 22 hospitals).
34. Excerpt from Chapter 3 (MeGadoRe Project, France).
35. Peter L, Straka P, Kovarova A, Kuca K, Maresova P. Regulatory issues in sustainable healthcare (Chapter 7).
36. FDA Artificial Intelligence. Machine learning in software as a medical device action plan. 2021. [online].

# Index





E. Ranschaert et al. (eds.), *Sustainability of AI in Radiology*, Imaging Informatics for Healthcare Professionals,
https://doi.org/10.1007/978-3-032-15693-8

**O**



**P**



**Q**



**R**



**S**



**T**

The manufacturer's authorised representative in the EU is Springer Nature Customer Service Centre GmbH, Europaplatz 3, 69115 Heidelberg, Germany. If you have any concerns regarding our products, please contact ProductSafety@springernature.com

Printed and bound by CPI Group (UK) Ltd, Croydon, CR0 4YY

12/07/2026

02164662-0001